Boomer's Guide to

Getting the Weight Off ... For Good

Boomer's Guide to Getting the Weight Off … For Good

Roberta Schwartz Wennik, M.S., R.D.

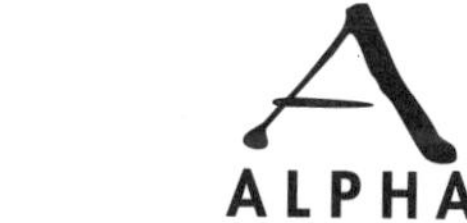

ALPHA
A member of Penguin Group (USA) Inc.

Copyright © 2003 by Roberta Schwartz Wennik

All rights reserved. No part of this book shall be reproduced, stored in a retrieval system, or transmitted by any means, electronic, mechanical, photocopying, recording, or otherwise, without written permission from the publisher. No patent liability is assumed with respect to the use of the information contained herein. Although every precaution has been taken in the preparation of this book, the publisher and author assume no responsibility for errors or omissions. Neither is any liability assumed for damages resulting from the use of information contained herein. For information, address Alpha Books, 800 East 96th Street, Indianapolis, IN 46240.

International Standard Book Number: 1-59257-160-3

Library of Congress Catalog Card Number: 2003112977

05 04 03 8 7 6 5 4 3 2 1

Interpretation of the printing code: The rightmost number of the first series of numbers is the year of the book's printing; the rightmost number of the second series of numbers is the number of the book's printing. For example, a printing code of 03-1 shows that the first printing occurred in 2003.

Printed in the United States of America

Note: This publication contains the opinions and ideas of its author. It is intended to provide helpful and informative material on the subject matter covered. It is sold with the understanding that the author and publisher are not engaged in rendering professional services in the book. If the reader requires personal assistance or advice, a competent professional should be consulted.

The author and publisher specifically disclaim any responsibility for any liability, loss, or risk, personal or otherwise, which is incurred as a consequence, directly or indirectly, of the use and application of any of the contents of this book.

Trademarks: All terms mentioned in this book that are known to be or are suspected of being trademarks or service marks have been appropriately capitalized. Alpha Books and Penguin Group (USA) Inc. cannot attest to the accuracy of this information. Use of a term in this book should not be regarded as affecting the validity of any trademark or service mark.

Most Alpha books are available at special quantity discounts for bulk purchases for sales promotions, premiums, fund-raising, or educational use. Special books, or book excerpts, can also be created to fit specific needs.

For details, write: Special Markets, Alpha Books, 375 Hudson Street, New York, NY 10014.

Publisher: Marie Butler-Knight
Product Manager: Phil Kitchel
Senior Managing Editor: Jennifer Chisholm
Senior Acquisitions Editor: Mike Sanders
Development Editor: Tom Stevens
Copy Editor: Keith Cline
Cover Designer: Doug Wilkins
Book Designer: Trina Wurst
Creative Director: Robin Lasek
Indexer: Brad Herriman
Layout/Proofreading: Angela Calvert, John Etchison

To Larry Wennik—my husband, my love and friend forever, and to my daughters, Debbie and Shari, and son-in-law, Scott, all who make my life infinitely complete.

Contents

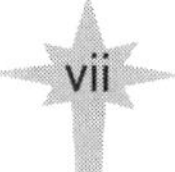

Introduction

You know you're a baby boomer if, when you were growing up …

- You wore saddle shoes (those white shoes with a black middle section). Tennis shoes or sneakers were our athletic shoes (because Nike and Adidas hadn't come into the consumer market yet). By the time we were teenagers, bell-bottom pants were in and tie-dye shirts were popular.
- You danced to the beat of The Beach Boys and The Beatles and tried doing the Twist.
- You owned a battery-operated transistor radio.
- You had to get up to change the television channels.
- The round disk you listened to was called a record, not a CD.
- You were glued to the television set as America witnessed Neil Armstrong become the first man to walk on the moon.

We "baby boomers" are a special group of people. I say "we" because I, too, am a baby boomer. Of course, you should never ask a lady her age, but suffice it to say, people called baby boomers were born between 1946 and 1964. We represent about 30 percent of the total population of the United States today. Our influence is so vast that media, television, and manufacturers of consumer products and foods vie for our attention and dollars. To some extent they helped foster our weight problem, and they're now supposedly trying to fix the problem. However, a weight problem is not so easily resolved with a simple diet product. It takes a permanent change of habits. That's where the *Boomer's Guide to Getting the Weight Off … For Good* will help you and will, hopefully, be all that you need to achieve your goals.

The Making of a Fat Generation

When we were growing up, a fat baby was considered a healthy baby because a fat body meant there was plenty to eat. Many of our parents had to sacrifice during World War II, so they didn't want to see their children go without, and overfeeding was not uncommon. Grandmothers seemed to love to pinch our chubby cheeks. We may have been chubby as babies, but most of us eventually slimmed down as children and adolescents. Spurred on by President Kennedy and his Council on Youth Fitness, physical education became a mandatory part of the school day. And we didn't yet have an addiction to television that would later turn us into couch potatoes. (With only five channels to choose from, there often wasn't anything interesting to watch anyway.) Because we didn't have computers and video games when we were growing up, we played outside.

Family and family values were important elements of the times. Sitting down together for breakfast and dinner were the norm. You actually took the time to dine, not wolf down your meal to go run off to do something else. After having gone without for so long during the war, women enjoyed setting a full table. For any child to leave anything on his or her plate was unthinkable. The memory of having had to live with so little was too fresh in the minds of many to let food go to waste. Therefore, children learned to "clean their plate," knowing that they wouldn't be excused from the table until they did.

That mind-set of cleaning our plate is very hard to break. If we hadn't yet been convinced to "make all gone," we were told about the many starving children in the world. How could we leave food on our plates when somewhere in the world a child had nothing to eat? (I wonder how many children fell for that, silently figuring that if they didn't eat what was on their plates, maybe they could just ship it over to those starving children?) This all might have contributed to the obesity we find in baby boomers today. It's not that we were necessarily fat children, but our minds had been programmed.

Jack LaLanne, the fitness guru of his time, took to the television airwaves in the late 1950s, showing us that fit is beautiful. He

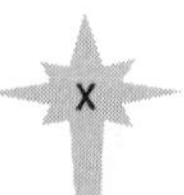

predated the likes of Richard Simmons and Jane Fonda by at least 25 years. I had the opportunity to interview him for my book *Your Personality Prescription,* when he shared with me how sad he thought it was to see how sedentary we boomers and our children had become. Here he was at 84 years old, still going strong, still challenging himself to be the best he could be. Why weren't we?

Laying Blame

The hippie generation, part of the baby boomer population, arose in the 1960s and 1970s. Hippies felt things needed to change from the restrictive and traditional ways of their parents. The influence of the hippies is still felt today. In fact, I believe some of our overweight problems are a result of the hippies believing "we can have it our way." (Makes you wonder if the ad campaign for Burger King with its slogan "Have it your way" was written by a boomer or to the boomers.) They believed we should all be free to follow our inner voices. Why listen to the authority figures, when all they wanted to do was deprive us of the good life? Maybe that's why baby boomers today don't like being told "you can't eat that" or "you must eat this." We want choices and the freedom to choose. "If I want to eat something or don't like to exercise, so what? It's my life. I'm free to choose."

Is technology to blame for our becoming overweight? We have remote controls so we don't have to get up to change the television channel. Dishwashers and washing machines have greatly reduced the calorie expenditure to get the job done. We have garage door openers that take a simple push of the button. If we humans can motorize something, we will (and become more inactive in the bargain)!

Maybe we can blame it on many households becoming two-income families. With the consequent affluence, it's possible to dine out more often. And as I'm sure you're aware, it's impossible to control the preparation (unless you're eating in a very cooperative restaurant) or the amount that is served. Fortunately, you do have control over how much you eat. We'll talk about that later. Our affluence shows in the number of packaged foods bought at the market. It's less expensive to make food from scratch, but fewer and fewer people want to take the time. It's more convenient to pop something into the oven (especially a microwave oven) and have dinner on the table in minutes. Clarence Birdseye, with his invention of frozen foods in waxed boxes, can probably take credit for setting us on the road to convenience foods. If it weren't for Birdseye, Minute Maid might never have processed oranges, condensing them and freezing the juice. This made orange juice more readily available to many parts of the United States. Swanson TV dinners might never have made their way into the freezer section. Mrs. Paul might never have made her fish sticks.

Television was a large influence on us—not just for the programming we saw, but for the meals we ate. With the television in the family room (as compared with today, where most households have a television in the kitchen), we needed TV trays and coffee tables to hold the TV dinners Swanson made for just this purpose. How convenient to just pop the tray in the oven and have no cleanup. Just throw away the container—the beginning of the disposable society and huge landfills. Food manufacturers took full advantage of this new love affair with the television, as they do today, selling us on foods we should try.

Watching television and eating at the same time might be part of the overweight problem we have today. Without fully focusing on what you're eating, you can eat far more than your body needs. How will you know when you've had enough? It's *not* when you've cleaned your plate or the TV program you've been watching is over!

Other food companies besides Swanson were vying for the family dollar. Kraft had its macaroni and cheese in a box. Campbell's Soups were used for casseroles. Franco-American offered up its SpaghettiOs for kids' lunches. Jell-O took convenience a step further when they introduced instant pudding that didn't have to be cooked. Hamburger Helper was glad to help rushed moms with their one-pot meals.

Convenience foods were becoming the staple of the American diet. At the time, no one questioned whether they were healthy, just that they were convenient. Do you remember the cartoon program on television called *The Jetsons?* It showed what life would be like in the twenty-first century. To prepare a meal, the family's robotic maid would simply push a button on what looked like an oven (called a Food-a-Rac-a-Cycle), and out came a complete meal. No refrigeration necessary. No preparation involved. Instant meal. If technology could come up with that one today, I'm sure there would be many buyers.

We might have eaten foods that were high in fat and sugar when we were growing up, but most of us were active enough to burn off those calories. Now that we're adults and less active, our problem might be that we're eating like we're still kids.

Dieting Might Have Made Us Fat—or at Least Kept Us That Way

Most people figure that the answer to the problem is to diet. However, dieting might either be causing the problem or fueling it. Look at the following figure to see what I mean. Let's assume you've put on "a few extra pounds." You want to lose weight to become thinner again, so you "go on a diet." At this point, we won't concern ourselves with what kind of diet, but just that it has fewer calories than you've been eating lately. By being forced to give up many of the foods you enjoy, you find yourself craving those foods. To show your body who's boss, you exert as much willpower as possible, only to find that, in time, your self-control begins to fade. The next thing you know, you're binging on the "outlawed" foods (feeling guilty, but at least satisfying your craving). Before you know it, you've gained back the weight (maybe even more than you lost), and you're ready to start the cycle again. The problem has not gone away. In fact, the problem is worse now, because you might have lost some self-esteem in the process. All you can see is that you've failed, or worse, that you're a failure.

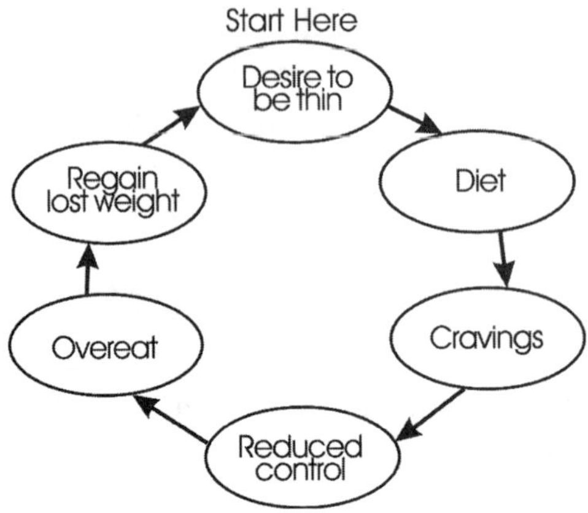

Dieter's cycle.

What has been called "yo-yo dieting" is basically going through the dieter's cycle numerous times, hoping that one of those times you'll lose the weight permanently and get off the merry-go-round. How many cycles do you have to go through before you realize that "dieting" doesn't work? *Boomer's Guide to Getting the Weight Off … For Good* isn't a diet, but a lifelong eating plan for health. As we were growing up, the focus of most diets was to get the weight off so you'd fit into your clothes. Those diets rarely emphasized the real value of losing weight—feeling more energetic, reducing your risk for the major diseases of heart disease, diabetes, and cancer, and feeling better about yourself. These are major factors for giving you a chance at more years to enjoy life, and enjoy it more fully.

Acknowledgments

To Larry Wennik, my husband, for his editing and research help on this book, the great discussions we had on what it means to be a boomer, and the many nights of washing dishes so I could go back to work to meet such a short book deadline.

To Mike Sanders, my editor, for giving me the opportunity to not only walk down memory lane and revisit many of the highlights of growing up as a boomer but also to help fellow boomers in their pursuit of health.

To Marilyn Allen, my agent, who served as matchmaker, connecting me with Mike Sanders to write a book that could potentially make a difference for those who need to lose weight.To Tom Stevens, Christy Wagner, and Keith Cline, three great editors, who helped set the standard for this exciting new series. Thanks for your attention to detail, meaning and flow.

part 1

Nutrition Class Is in Session

The essentials of good nutrition haven't changed all that much since we were younger. The concepts of eating your vegetables, having variety in your meals, and eating in moderation have been around for many more years than we are old. Didn't your mother tell you to "eat your vegetables or you won't get dessert"? Throughout our lifetime, science has delved into understanding the effects of nutrition on our health. In turn, health professionals and educators have tried to translate this new scientific information into something usable for the consumer. Having the knowledge of what makes for good nutrition puts you in the driver's seat, being able to make the appropriate decisions on what to eat. Therefore, in this section I share with you a Boomer's Guide Food Pyramid, a way to select your fruits and vegetables, a reminder to be sure that fiber is in your diet, how to take the fear out of fat, and lastly, how to find room for dessert. Let's not forget that even Mom said we could have dessert!

chapter 1

Sabotaging Yourself

Conscience is the inner voice warning us that someone may be looking.

—H. L. Mencken

People sabotage their desire and efforts to lose weight in many ways. See if any of these sounds like what you've done in the past. I'd rather have you address them now, before you get started on the *Boomer's Guide to Getting the Weight Off … For Good* because I very much want you to be successful. I also really want this to be the last time you have to lose weight or think of yourself as a heavy person. The picture I have for you is that, by the time you've finished reading this book, you'll have found the perfect method that works for you, learned more about what it means to be a healthy person, and made plans to stay that way.

The Who in You

Are you a perfectionist? If so, what happens when you eat something you feel you shouldn't have eaten or when you don't get around to exercising? Do you get upset with yourself? In trying to lose weight, perfectionism can cause stress if the goals you've set aren't achieved—or aren't achieved on time. Perfectionists have many *shoulds* in their lives. Yet, it's often hard to be perfect every day. Inevitably, something will come up that will interfere. Because you're a perfectionist, you may want to punish yourself for messing up. You may do something irrational, like not eating the next day to make up for the overindulgence. Or you may exercise twice as long and hard for having missed an exercise session—this isn't the worst idea, unless you set yourself up for injury in the process. Or you may just binge. The best thing to do is just get right back on track, realizing that one mishap is not going to prevent you from achieving your goal. Progress is more important than perfection.

Are you an idealist? If you're an idealist, you're in even worse shape than the perfectionist. You tend to set such lofty goals that achieving them is next to impossible. In some cases, those goals aren't even realistic. And even if you do achieve them, you'll probably reset them even higher, thinking that you probably set the original goal too low. In many ways, it's because you never let yourself feel satisfied. Because of that, you never stop to reward yourself for your accomplishments. Staying in the present moment would help—that way you can view what happened today as worthwhile, and not worry that you haven't yet reached the lofty goals you've set.

Do you tend to follow what your heart feels rather than what your head is telling you? If someone baked a cake for your birthday, but your diet plan doesn't allow for high-calorie desserts (or you hadn't planned for those calories by eating lower-calorie foods during the day), would you eat it? Some people wouldn't think of hurting the baker's feelings, after the baker was so nice to do something special for them. Or do you make foods to satisfy the eating desires of others, knowing that partaking of those foods may cause you to go over your daily calorie and fat allowances? It may be sabotaging your weight-loss efforts, but you don't want to hurt anyone else's feelings. All the while, your head is telling you that you're doing in your weight-loss efforts. Does your head win out or does your heart?

Are you one of those the "diet-starts-Monday-morning" people? This is just another form of procrastinating. Many people use it as an excuse to eat, drink, and be merry over the weekend, thinking that they'll do penance and atone starting Monday morning. Do you realize what kind of mind-set you're going into a diet with when you think this way? From that perspective, dieting is punishment for having gotten fat. Instead of thinking of losing weight as a way of becoming healthier and having more energy, something that should be positive, losing weight is the sentence handed down on you and your life. I'd rather have you say "today is the first day of the rest of my life." Why wait until Monday? Unless, of course, today happens to be Monday!

Are you a "what-might-be" kind of person? Do you tend to lose track of the details of what it takes every day to reach your goal? Seeing where you're headed (your vision or goal) is very helpful in pulling you forward toward your weight-loss goals. However, if you focus too much on the future, and neglect what you have to do today to lose that weight, you may never reach your goal. The problem with looking too far into the future is that it gives you too much slack in what you do today. The future is anything you want it to be—but today is reality. It's very much like being a member of the "diet-starts-Monday-morning" club.

Do you want to lose weight, but find yourself putting it off? Maybe you're hoping to find the best way to lose weight, one that can guarantee results (instant results, actually). Or maybe you always have something else that takes precedence. Do you think you're a procrastinator, wanting to lose weight, but always finding some reason you can't get started? While you might have been quick to decide to lose weight, actually getting started is a whole lot harder. There's a saying in the technology field that applies handily here. You should keep this in mind when you find yourself still in the planning phase. "It's time to shoot the engineer and get the process into production." Engineers are perfectionists, who feel that, given more time, they can make whatever they're working on better. However, there comes a time when taking action is more valuable than improving the plans just a little bit more.

Are you an "I've-got-to-see-it-to-believe-it" kind of person? If this describes you, what will be your reaction when you're following all the rules to lose weight and nothing's happening? Maybe you were able to take off the first couple of pounds quickly, but for all your efforts, you feel you've stalled—you're going nowhere fast. Will you be tempted to ditch the diet and go back to life as it was? Remember, if you decide to go this route, you're no closer to being healthier or having more energy than when you started. And I can't imagine that giving up is going to do anything positive for your self-esteem and ego.

Are you afraid to lose weight because you can't see yourself as a thin person? Sometimes people may sabotage the weight-loss effort because they don't internally see themselves as being a slim person, just a heavy person wanting to be slim. Changing your image of yourself needs to come first, before you can take action.

Goal Getter

Do you find that starting a new diet is exciting? Do you have an initial sense of anticipation and hopefulness, only to find that your enthusiasm wanes in a short time? At the beginning, isn't it like being a child again? Do you remember getting a toy and wanting to play with it over and over, and telling everyone about it? But, sooner or later, you were off doing something else, forgetting completely about the toy. Furthermore, if you're an optimist, you probably believe, and have said to yourself, that this time this diet is going to work. The fact that you're willing to start another new diet means that you still believe in yourself. And that self-belief is such an important part of being successful at anything you do. However, you'll need to keep a close watch on yourself to make sure that you don't give up on your enthusiasm as you near the end. Or that you lose your enthusiasm because you're getting bored with the process. The longer it takes, the further away you get from that first excitement of getting started. If this is going to be your way of life, you'd better not get bored with it.

Do you find that you goal-set *to* your goal and not *through* your goal? Even though you may not want to admit it, losing weight and maintaining a healthy level is a forever project. We're not yet that old, boomers, but as we do get older, our bodies will want to hold more fat. Think of weight management as just one of the many chores you have in your life that you just do—like brushing your teeth every day.

Do you ever see yourself not brushing your teeth every day? Then why should watching your weight have a set time frame or stop when you no longer have extra pounds to be concerned with? That would be the same thing as no longer brushing your teeth because your dentist told you on your last exam that you had no cavities.

Do you set goals that are too large and unrealistic? Do they tend to be so out of reach that you're so intimidated by the challenge that you quit before you even get started? For example, someone who has 75 to 100 pounds to lose may feel that this is too overwhelming a job to do. Setting short-term goals may work better to get you going. When I tell myself that all I have to lose in the first step is 25 pounds, I can picture myself being able to do that. After I've succeeded at doing that once, I have no excuse for not going for another 25 pounds. I already know that I can be successful. And depending on how much weight you want to lose, you can use any appropriate first chunk. So, again for example, if you want to lose 25 pounds, you might make the first chunk 10 or 15 pounds. For those of you who like the "new beginnings," setting smaller goals means you get to start fresh every so many pounds.

Seeing Results

Do you set too short a time frame for accomplishing your goals? Do you set yourself up to expect results in an unreasonable amount of time? I figure that if I'm changing my lifestyle habits for good, there really isn't any need for a time frame, other than a lifetime. If I'm doing all that I can do to eat healthfully, and I'm exercising as much as I can or want to, then the results will speak for themselves. All I can get are the results I get. Setting a time frame only puts pressure on me that cannot have a hold on me forever. So when the pressure, or my response to it, wears off, so does the motivation. Some people work better under pressure because they think it makes them more committed to accomplishing the goal. Take for example someone losing weight for a class reunion that's coming up in five months. That's just enough pressure to get things done—maybe. Let's remember, though, that that's a goal being set *to,* not *through.* What do you think is going to happen once the reunion has come and gone?

Do you continue to do the same thing over and over but expect different results? If you haven't had success on a diet, do you try it again—figuring this time it will work? What if the plan isn't right for you? Maybe you've gotten involved in an exercise program and you're lifting weights. If you started out on 2- or 3-pound weights, are you still using the same amount of weight and expecting to see better results? Something has to change. This can even apply to how you think about dieting. If you think that dieting is a temporary measure to lose weight, following which you can go back to your old lifestyle habits, how do you think you'll end up? You're obviously going to gain the weight back. How many times do you have to repeat this cycle before you realize that, unless you make a permanent change in your lifestyle, you have no right to expect different results?

Do you blame others for your being overweight or for you not having success losing weight? The favorite line of most people is "it's my genes." Another one is "my folks forced me to clean my plate and now I can't stop." "It's my friend's birthday and I had to have a piece of cake—it's bad luck not to." "My kids want to have treats in the house, and I can't resist them (the treats *and* the kids)." The blame game gets you no closer to your goal.

Do you expect immediate results, even though it took you years to become heavy? Somehow, people figure that if they change the way they're eating and start doing some exercising, they should immediately look thinner and the scale should give them some happy news. Because you didn't become overweight overnight, you shouldn't expect to lose it overnight. Having an expectation like that is just setting you up for quitting.

Do you tend to give up too quickly? Part of the reason people give up too quickly is because their expectations for immediate results aren't fulfilled (and couldn't be). Another reason is that what they have to do isn't enjoyable and feels like punishment. That's where many people make the mistake. They don't take the time to find an approach that feels right to them; so instead, they end up having to use willpower to make the program they're on work for them. Because the experience isn't enjoyable, they feel "the quicker I can get out of this, the better." Because willpower doesn't last very long, many people give up.

The Eating Experience

Do you find that you eat more when you're with others? Studies have shown that people tend to eat more than they should when they're socializing with others. Worse yet, the amount of food that's eaten is directly related to the number of people in the group—the more people, the more food consumed. There are several possible explanations. One is that we tend to linger over our food longer when there are others eating. Another is that, with lots of conversation, it's difficult to focus on what and how much you're eating. Some people love to socialize so much that they'll find every excuse in the book to get together. In the United States, and some other parts of the world, eating is an important part of socializing.

As you're eating your main course, are you already thinking about dessert? If this is typical for you, then you're not focusing on your food. You can't really be thinking about the flavors and textures of what you're eating when your mind is somewhere else (like the dessert course).

Do you eat dinner while watching television or reading a book? If this is you, then I don't know how you can really appreciate the flavors of the meal or know when you've eaten enough. If you want to watch television or read, go sit on the sofa (without food). I know we boomers were raised on TV dinners and the concept of watching television while eating. However, it's just not a good idea. Besides, with as little time as families have to spend together, sitting down to a meal and enjoying each other's company can be far more valuable than watching television. It's a great opportunity to share the day's events. That reminds me of when my girls were younger and I'd ask them, as they arrived home from school, what had happened in their day. Their usual response was, "Oh, nothing." Yet as we sat at the dinner table and had a peaceful time to talk, all the exciting things that had happened to them that day spilled out, without any prompting. When I think back on my years growing up as a boomer, I still like the image on the television show *Father Knows Best* of everyone sitting around the table talking about this or that. I just wish more people still honored this tradition.

Do you tend to eat when you're under stress? Stress can cause a person to act out of character, giving up responsibility for personal weight management. Instead of food being a source of nourishment, it's used to provide comfort. The choice of foods may "go against the rules," potentially being high in calories and fat. Do you remember how certain foods seemed to console you in the past? When you're under stress, do you look to those same foods for comfort? If that's what you're doing, it should make you stop and think about what's causing you the stress. Deal with the stress directly, rather than through food.

Are you an impulsive eater? Given the opportunity, will you accept an eating invitation because it sounds like fun? When you're trying to lose weight, responding to every enticement to eat isn't going to get you closer to your goal. What if you're not hungry? Will you eat anyway? If someone brought Krispy Kreme doughnuts into work, would you be able to pass them by or would they call too loudly to you to be ignored?

chapter 2

Look How Far Good Nutrition Has Come

Food is an important part of a balanced diet.
—Fran Lebowitz

More than 2,000 years ago, the pharaohs of Egypt had their architects build them pyramids for burial chambers. Time has proven the pyramid to be a very stable structure. This is primarily due to a broad base that easily supports its upper layers. Keep that in mind when we start talking about why the United States Department of Agriculture (USDA) chose this shape as the design for the Food Guide Pyramid and, in turn, how we can use it to construct a healthy diet.

For many years, the USDA has collected data on food consumption patterns, food composition, cost of food, and the nutritional status of Americans. One of the USDA's jobs is to translate all this information into dietary recommendations that Americans can use to stay healthy. The Food Guide Pyramid is the result.

A Bit of History

The Food Guide Pyramid is not the first effort by the USDA to provide recommendations for Americans. There have been food guidelines as far back as 1894. At that time, there was a concern about nutritional deficiencies (as compared to today, where we now must be concerned with overabundance).

From 1894 to 1940, the government put its energies into instructing Americans on how to feed their children well so we would have a strong and healthy population. Booklets with such titles as "Good Food Habits" and "Good Proportions in the Diet" were published to help mothers with these issues.

During World War II, the government was still encouraging Americans to eat well, this time for the war cause. The slogan was "U.S. Needs US Strong—Eat Nutritional Foods." However, with many foods being scarce, the government tried to make suggestions about appropriate substitutions and provided guidelines known as the "Daily 8" for eating well.

The Daily 8
(Food Guidelines from the USDA in 1943)

Here's how to grow strong, America—eat these foods every day:

- Milk and milk products—at least a pint for everyone—more for children—or cheese or evaporated milk or dried milk
- Bread and cereal—whole-grain products or enriched bread and flour
- Oranges, tomatoes, grapefruit or raw cabbage or salad green—at least one of these
- Meat, poultry, or fish—dry beans, peas, or nuts occasionally
- Green or yellow vegetables—one big helping or more—some raw, some cooked
- Eggs—at least 3 or 4 a week, cooked any way you choose—or in "made" dishes
- Other vegetables, fruits—potatoes, other vegetables, or fruits in season
- Butter and other spreads—vitamin-rich fats, peanut butter, and similar spreads
- Then eat other foods you like, too.

They even made recommendations as to the number of servings that would be appropriate. Notice in the Daily 8 there was attention paid to the color of the fruits and vegetables we were encouraged to eat. As you will see, the government eventually dropped the distinction in the color of the fruits and vegetables as separate food categories. That's unfortunate, because research today is finding that the color of the foods you eat has a major impact on your health.

> Back in the nineteenth and early twentieth centuries, obesity was not a national issue.

From the end of the war until 1955, the USDA decided to combine fruits into one group of foods and vegetables into another, reducing the number of food categories from eight to seven. Instead of the food guide being in the shape of the pyramid we have today, the USDA used a circle divided into wedges to show us the various food categories. At that time, there was no intent to show the relative amounts of food from each category by the size of the wedges, which were all equal. It was just a pictorial representation of the different food groups:

- Milk
- Vegetables
- Fruits
- Eggs
- Meat, cheese, fish, and poultry
- Cereal and bread
- Butter

The government did make suggestions as to the minimum amounts that should be eaten from each group. You have to remember that we were still in a "promote eating" mentality. These guidelines were an attempt to ensure that people received at least a minimum of nutrition. Today's Food Guide Pyramid provides the maximum number of servings. The message from the government now is "there is a healthy limit."

The Four Food Groups

From 1955 to 1979, the seven categories were reduced to four. It's not that certain foods didn't need to be eaten. It's just that the government was trying to simplify things by combining fruits and vegetables into one category, putting eggs in the meat group, and eliminating butter as a separate food group. The importance of butter in the diet was demoted.

The USDA called this new set of four food groups "Food for Fitness—A Daily Food Guide." The concept of fitness had now become a new part of the government's objective in nutritional recommendations.

In 1979, the USDA introduced the "Hassle-Free Daily Food Guide." In addition to the four food groups, it added a fifth one—fats, sweets, and alcohol—with a warning to use with caution, moderating one's intake of these. It also shared what a serving consisted of. For example, a serving of bread was one slice, and a serving of milk was one cup. The USDA was acknowledging the fact that more homemakers and mothers were entering the workforce. Considering how little time they had to prepare food, they needed easy-to-follow guidelines for serving their families a healthy meal. As I mentioned earlier, the food manufacturers were more than willing to help the cause by providing packaged foods, even if they weren't always the healthiest.

> **The People's Choice for the Four Food Groups**
>
> *Choice A:* Chocolate candy, chocolate ice cream, chocolate pudding, and chocolate cake
>
> *Choice B:* Junk food, fast food, frozen food, and spoiled food
>
> *Choice C:* Canned, frozen, catered, and takeout
>
> And the winner is …

By the 1980s, the USDA wasn't just using food consumption and food composition data to determine healthy guidelines. It was using studies of the relationship of food intake to the risk of diseases. One particular study that drew a great deal of attention was the Framingham Heart Study that began in 1948. By studying people like our parents, they were establishing data that they hoped would serve future generations. By the time the last of us baby boomers had been born (about the early

1960s), the Framingham researchers had discovered that factors such as high blood cholesterol, smoking, high blood pressure, and obesity increased one's risk for heart disease. With all this evidence, the government needed to be more aggressive in its recommendations to the American public.

The Dietary Guidelines

The first edition of the "Dietary Guidelines for Americans" came out in 1980. Its wording tended more toward "avoid this and avoid that." The government was no longer concerned about nutrient deficiencies, considering that the level of obesity was rising. Feedback through the years since the first edition told the USDA that we baby boomers didn't want to hear all that negative rhetoric. We wanted it more positive. Therefore, in the 2000 edition, the wording had been changed to "choose this and select this in moderation." The latest edition (the fifth edition, released in 2000) tries to make the guidelines appealing by putting the 10 guidelines under three major messages called the "ABCs for Good Health—**A**im for fitness, **B**uild a healthy base, and **C**hoose sensibly."

When aiming for fitness: (1) Aim for a healthy weight and (2) be physically active each day.

To build a healthy base: (1) Let the pyramid guide your food choices; (2) choose a variety of grains daily, especially whole grains; (3) choose a variety of fruits and vegetables daily; and (4) keep food safe to eat.

When choosing sensibly: (1) Choose a diet that is low in saturated fat and cholesterol and moderate in total fat; (2) choose beverages and foods to moderate your intake of sugars; (3) choose and prepare foods with less salt; and (4) if you drink alcoholic beverages, do so in moderation.

The Food Guide Pyramid Is Born

The Food Guide Pyramid was a natural follow-on piece to the "Dietary Guidelines" because Americans needed something to help them implement the guidelines. And it served as a good visual reference.

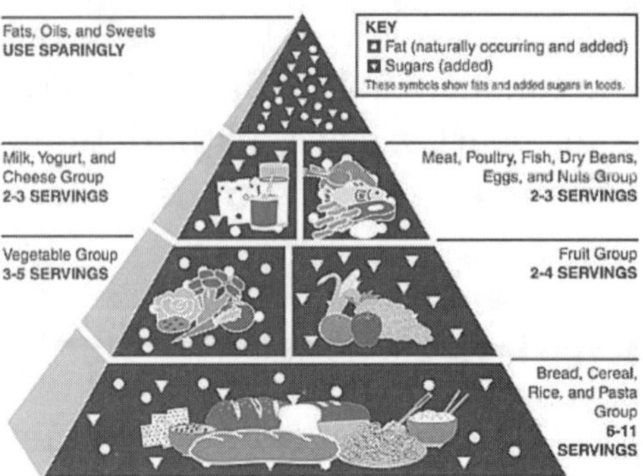

USDA Food Guide Pyramid.

It definitely was a big step forward from the four food groups. Because the Food Guide Pyramid is based on the "Dietary Guidelines," it takes into consideration the relationship of nutrition and the major diseases, something that wasn't a concern of the four food groups. In some cases, the nutrient composition of a food determines in what group it's placed on the pyramid. Legumes and dried beans are included in the meat group because they are high in protein. (They're also high in carbohydrates and could just have easily gone in the starch group.) However, there are some foods that are placed where one would naturally think to find them. Good examples are the potato and corn. While they are placed in the vegetable group, with their being so much higher in carbohydrates than other vegetables, they would more appropriately fit in the starch group. (So for those of you who want to say you had your vegetables by eating a potato or corn, think again. I believe I've finally convinced my meat-and-potatoes son-in-law of that.)

A great deal of research went into the design of the Food Guide Pyramid. There were suggestions of using the design of a plate or a bowl instead of a pyramid to display the food groups. The beauty of the pyramid shape is that it provides a vehicle for showing us how we can eat a variety of foods by selecting items from different food groups. It also shows us how to apply proportionality to the amount of food we eat, based on the relative sizes of the food groups on the pyramid. Lastly, because the tip of the pyramid is so small, we learn to use moderation when eating foods high in fat and sugar.

The proportionality aspect of the pyramid is important to consider. Each food group's contribution to the overall diet is represented by its placement on the pyramid. Just as having a broad base has allowed the Egyptian pyramids to stand through all these years, so should our diets have the broad base of grains and complex carbohydrates. Advocates of high-protein diets may argue that point. That debate continues to raise voices on both sides.

As we proceed up the Food Guide Pyramid, we can see that the next two big contributors to our diet are fruits and vegetables. When we were growing up, the four food groups combined fruits and vegetables into one category. If you didn't like vegetables, this was a good deal. You could satisfy that food group by eating just fruit. With so much research pointing to the health value of certain phytochemicals (plant chemicals) found in vegetables (but not found in fruit), we can no longer ignore our vegetables. Based on this research, the USDA reverted to their previous thinking and divided the group back into separate food groups.

The challenge with any tool like the Food Guide Pyramid is that it must address the needs of many people. That's why there is a range of servings based on how many calories someone of your age, sex, size, and activity level should have. The USDA used three calorie levels:

- 1,600 calories for many sedentary women and some older adults
- 2,200 calories for most children, teenage girls, active women, and many sedentary men (women who are pregnant or breastfeeding may need a bit more)
- 2,800 calories for teenage boys, active men, and some very active women

In the early part of 2003, the Food Guide Pyramid came under attack in such magazines as *Newsweek* and *Scientific American.* The articles said that the Food Guide Pyramid was crumbling. With Americans getting fatter and fatter, the pyramid was not solving the problem. In fact, they blamed the pyramid for causing the obesity epidemic, saying that our search for a low-fat diet put too much emphasis on carbohydrates. The writers of the articles ignored the fact that the average American isn't eating according to the pyramid. Many of the carbohydrates

Americans are eating aren't whole grains, but sweets. Furthermore, the portion sizes Americans are choosing to eat are far larger than those recommended on the Food Guide Pyramid. Chapters 11 and 12 review the opinions of the opposition to the Food Guide Pyramid.

chapter 3

Variations on a Pyramid Theme

Tomatoes and oregano make it Italian; wine and tarragon make it French. Lemon and cinnamon make it Greek ... garlic makes it good.

—Alice May Brock

Because the Food Guide Pyramid is such a powerful design, many look-alikes have come along. There are pyramids that have been adapted for kids, vegetarians, and ethnic and cultural groups. Among the many versions of the Food Guide Pyramid, the most interesting, and for some the most controversial, is the Mediterranean Diet Pyramid. It was created based on the dietary habits of the people from the Mediterranean region, where olive oil reigns supreme as the dietary fat of choice and red meat is eaten only as an occasional treat. With America's love affair with beef, eating meat as a treat isn't likely to happen soon. However, keep your minds open. We're going to take a closer look at the Mediterranean Diet Pyramid to see if it gives any hints as to why these people have a lower risk of chronic disease and a greater life expectancy than Americans. There may be some lessons to learn.

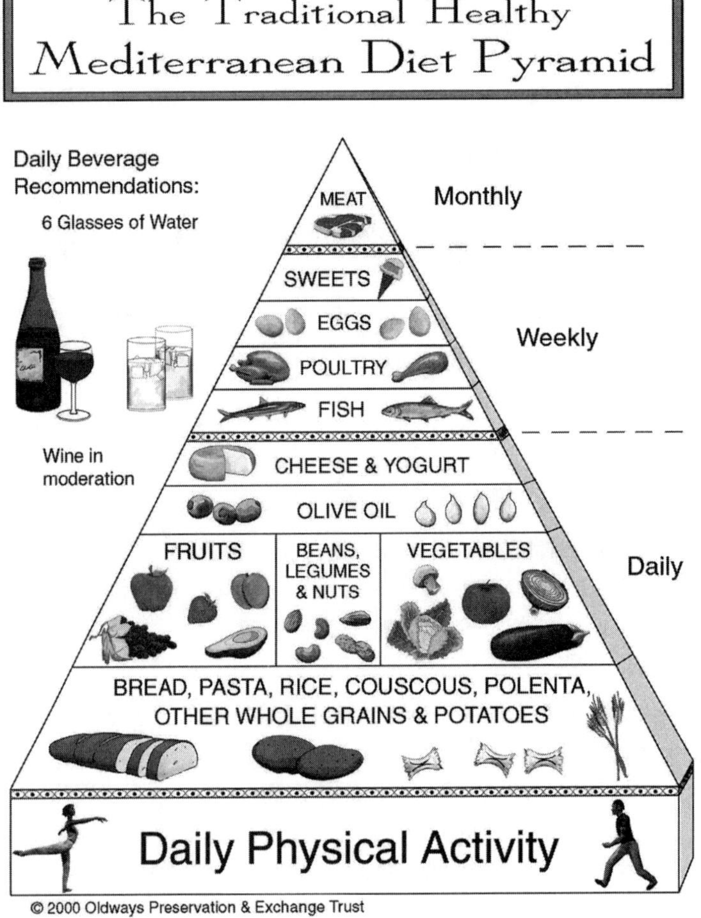

Mediterranean Diet Pyramid.

A Call to Action

You'll notice that the Mediterranean Diet Pyramid includes daily physical activity at its base—a good reminder to all that activity contributes to overall good health. Even though the USDA "Dietary Guidelines" discuss physical activity, it's unfortunate that the USDA Food Guide

Pyramid doesn't share this message in its design as we see with the Mediterranean Diet Pyramid. When you consider that more people are familiar with the Food Guide Pyramid than the "Dietary Guidelines," this is a lost opportunity. You now have been given a heads-up. Get active.

The amount of daily physical activity is one major difference between the lifestyles of Americans and the Mediterranean people. Americans have become a very sedentary group, what with all the modern technological innovations that have occurred during our lifetime. My mother used to own a scrubboard, even though she did have a washing machine. Many clothes just needed some heavy-duty cleaning. Washing machines today take care of the ground-in dirt. We had a dryer, but she often hung the clothes out on a clothesline to dry. When I was growing up, airports didn't have walking conveyor belts to whisk you quickly to the terminals. The television remote control didn't exist. We actually had to get up to change the television channel. I could go on about the many conveniences we baby boomers now have that didn't exist as we were growing up. Those conveniences are nice, but they're doing us in.

It's not that the Mediterranean people don't have conveniences. However, they generally tend to do more walking and less driving than we do. They don't tend do their grocery shopping on a weekly basis. They'll stop by their local market for the night's dinner ingredients and then walk home. They use more public transportation, which requires them to walk to a pickup point.

Is It Animal or Vegetable?

Both pyramids have grains, vegetables, and fruits at the bottom, providing a nice solid base to our diets. The differences become obvious the higher up we go on the pyramids. Because the Mediterranean Diet Pyramid is largely a vegetarian diet, it recommends people eat animal protein such as fish, poultry, and eggs only once a week and limit meat to once a month. The Food Guide Pyramid, on the other hand, supports eating from all the food groups on a daily basis.

The problem with the Mediterranean Diet Pyramid suggesting animal protein be limited to one serving a week is that animal protein is a good source of iron and zinc, nutrients women are often lacking. You can include animal protein in your diet as long as you select lean cuts, which have less of the unhealthy saturated fat.

I like the fact that the Mediterranean Diet Pyramid assigns separate sections to the different sources of protein. Fish, poultry, eggs, and meat each have their own box. It makes us aware that these foods contribute to our diets in different ways. I wish the Food Guide Pyramid did the same thing. By the Food Guide Pyramid grouping animal and vegetable sources of protein together, all are given equal weight without distinction to their impact on the risk of disease.

I told you in the last chapter that foods in the Food Guide Pyramid are placed, in most cases, into particular categories based on their nutrient composition. That is why the meat group contains animal proteins (meat, poultry, fish, and eggs) and plant proteins (dry beans, *legumes*, and nuts).

They all are good sources of protein. The problem is they differ widely in their fat, cholesterol, and fiber content. Beans, legumes, and nuts don't have any cholesterol, and they have plenty of fiber. (I know, occasionally that tough piece of beef tastes like it has plenty of fiber! But it doesn't.) With Americans not getting enough fiber, making beans, legumes, and nuts a separate food group would be a good idea. It would visually suggest we increase our intake of them.

What's a Legume?

Legumes and dry peas are close relatives to the dry bean. Some common legumes include lentils, dry peas, soybeans, and chickpeas. Legumes have been around for thousands of years and have served as a good source of protein. When you're having pinto, kidney, or lima beans, you're having dry beans. Have a bowl of split pea soup or a dish of chili and get a good helping of fiber.

A Food Group Just for Olive Oil

Olive oil has a separate grouping in the Mediterranean Diet Pyramid. By making it an individual section, you get the sense of its importance. Being a monounsaturated fat, it is heart-healthy. It doesn't raise LDL (low-density lipoprotein) cholesterol, the bad form of cholesterol in the blood that can clog your vessels or lower the good HDL (high-density lipoprotein) cholesterol that helps the body sweep out some of the LDL cholesterol.

When we were younger, you could only get olive oil at specialty stores. Now most grocery stores stock at least one brand, if not more. There is a variety of flavors of olive oil, from the mild to those with peppery overtones. Be adventurous and experiment. Some delis will often give samples, which is always the best way to decide what to buy. At least, you can do a comparison of several types without committing to buying any particular one until you're sure you like it.

An Olive Oil Suggestion

Instead of putting margarine or butter on your bread, consider dipping it in a little bit of olive oil and balsamic vinegar.

There are other good sources of monounsaturated fats, including canola oil. It's not surprising that olive oil would occupy its own space on the Mediterranean Diet Pyramid, what with the Mediterranean region being the largest producer of the world's olive oil supply. The Food Guide Pyramid, on the other hand, only tells you to "use fats sparingly." What's "sparingly"? No mention is made of what fats are good to eat. (Check out Chapter 7 to find out more.)

The Best of Both Worlds

Both the Food Guide Pyramid and the Mediterranean Diet Pyramid are good attempts at getting people to eat better. The Food Guide Pyramid encourages people to eat more fruits and vegetables by recommending the number of servings and placing these groups on the bottom half of the design. The Mediterranean Diet Pyramid supports eating more fish, a good source of the heart-protective fatty acid called omega-3 and selecting olive oil for fat. It also appreciates that potatoes are high in starch, and even though we call them vegetables, they are better placed in the starch group at the base of the pyramid. Another difference between the Food Guide Pyramid and the Mediterranean Diet Pyramid involves where to place cheese. The Food Guide Pyramid puts it in the milk, yogurt, and cheese group because it is a great source of calcium. Yet, the nutrient breakdown of cheese makes it more like meat. It is basically protein and fat with very little carbohydrate.

I personally believe there would be value in combining the two pyramids into something like the following where you get the best of both worlds. I'm calling it the Boomer's Guide Pyramid. (I have not included number of servings because that will be tailored for you in Part 3.)

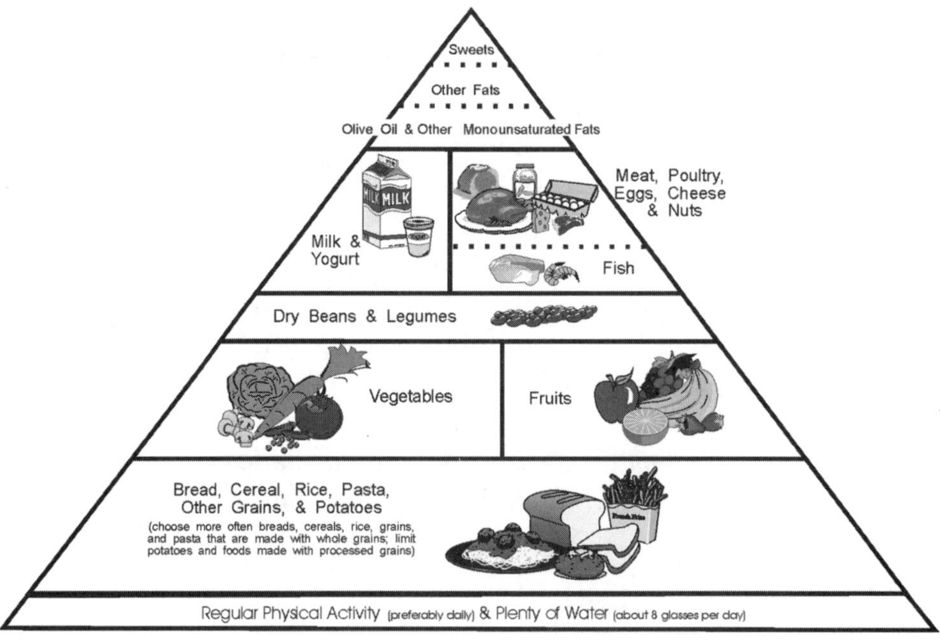

Boomer's Guide Pyramid.

There's an emphasis on eating fish at least one to two times per week as your protein source; dry beans and legumes eaten daily give you a good source of fiber, protein, and carbohydrates with little fat. Olive oil and other monounsaturated fats (such as canola oil) are highlighted, so that when fat is eaten, these healthier choices will be considered.

We should keep the pyramid in mind as we make food selections. Are we picking too many foods from one group and ignoring another group? I don't know about you, but I'm a visual person, where "a picture is worth a thousand words." I like to keep the image of the pyramid in my mind when making food selections, trying to be sure to choose from each of the groups, except maybe the "other fats" and "sweets." Those are not mandatory foods. Of course, someone with a sweet tooth might say otherwise!

chapter 4

Brought to You in Living Color

The next time you feel like complaining, remember that your garbage disposal probably eats better than 30 percent of the people in the world.

—Robert Orben

Mother Nature works very hard for us, producing a bounty of food in an exciting array of colors. From her luscious red tomatoes to vibrant orange cantaloupes, her color palette would make any artist *green* with envy. Yet the average American plate is filled with the boring beige of french fries, the dark brown of ground beef, and the insipid green of iceberg lettuce. Does your plate need a color makeover?

Have you ever wondered why there are so many different colored fruits and vegetables? The colors tell you a lot about what nutrients these foods contain. In fact, the deeper and richer the color, the greater the amount of nutrients. For example, when buying cabbage, find the greener heads. Only now are scientists beginning to unravel what those nutrients and chemicals are and what possible benefits they offer. When you and I were young, scientists understood that vegetables and fruits held a powerhouse of nutrients. They were just starting to look deep within foods for the nutrition they held, and in turn, the affect on the body. You can see that the color of food was important even back in 1943, when the USDA created the Daily 8 food guidelines. Green and yellow vegetables were in a food group of their own.

Yet it wasn't until the 1970s that scientists started piecing together the puzzle and realizing that plants held not only vitamins and minerals, but other chemicals that are now called *phytochemicals.* In the 1980s and 1990s, there was more intense study to try to "mine" fruits and vegetables for their chemical properties. It was hoped that these chemicals could eventually be made into medicines or what were dubbed *nutriceuticals* or included in manufactured foods called *functional foods.*

> The term *phyto* comes from the Greek word for "plant."

Phytochemicals are naturally occurring substances found in fruits, vegetables, legumes, whole grains, seeds, herbs, and tea. They contribute to the flavor, the color, and the plant's own resistance to disease. Research is showing that phytochemicals have health-promoting potential, especially in their ability to decrease your risk of cancer, scavenge free radicals (molecules that can be destructive to the body), strengthen blood vessel walls, interfere with processes that lead to heart disease and stroke, and boost your immune response.

Optimal levels for phytochemicals have yet to be determined. In fact, the field of phytochemicals is still in its infancy, with only a handful of chemicals having been identified.

Because foods that contain phytochemicals also contain vitamins, minerals and fiber, it's smart to include these in your diet. *That means eating plenty of fruits and vegetables.* Another plus is that these foods, in most cases, are fairly low in calories and fat—when eaten in their natural state. So please don't think that eating a slice of apple pie is the same as eating a raw apple, for example.

How Many Fruits and Vegetables Are You Eating?

Although the Food Guide Pyramid suggests eating three to five servings of vegetables a day, along with two to four servings of fruit, most Americans aren't even coming close. The consumption data available from the government lumps fruits and vegetables together as part of the National Cancer Institute's 5-a-Day for Better Health program. If the number of servings of fruits and vegetables recommended on the pyramid were grouped together, you'd have to eat a *minimum* of five servings a day. Looking at the data from the USDA's "Continuing Surveys of Food Intakes by Individuals (CSFII)" for the year 2000, the percentage of the population eating five or more servings of fruits and vegetables is as follows:

- 23.1 percent of the population nationwide
- 20 to 25 percent of the baby boomers
- 26.9 percent of women and 18.9 percent of men

People who were more active ate more fruits and vegetables. Compared to data from previous surveys, we are doing better than we used to. However, we're still a long way off from getting the protection that eating enough fruits and vegetables would give us. When you consider that the boomer population comprises the largest percentage of the overall population, we're not doing too well in the fruit and vegetable department. I can hear some of you saying, "But there aren't many vegetables I like." My response to that is "You're not looking hard enough." I'll admit that most of us grew up on carrot and celery sticks for lunch and maybe green beans for dinner, a banana for breakfast and an apple for lunch, but there's too much variety available today to say there's nothing you like.

With So Many Choices, No Excuses

It's not that we have to plant the fruits and vegetables ourselves, as our ancestors did. Most large modern supermarkets offer an astounding variety. Many areas of the United States are fortunate to not only get local produce, but also fruits and vegetables from other parts of the world. There is usually more space allotted to the produce department of a grocery store than any other department.

By the 1980s, a new group of produce was arriving on the scene—organically grown. For those of us not trusting that regular-grown produce was pesticide-free, we were turning to the organically grown, even though it was, and still is, more expensive. Standards have been set by the USDA to assure the public that they're getting what they pay for. According to the USDA, organic food is produced by farmers who emphasize the use of renewable resources and the conservation of soil and water to enhance environmental quality for future generations. It is supposed to be produced without using most conventional pesticides, fertilizers made with synthetic ingredients or sewage sludge, bioengineering, or ionizing radiation. Before a product can be labeled "organic," a government-approved certifier inspects the farm where the food is grown to make sure the farmer is following all the rules necessary to meet USDA organic standards. Companies that handle or process organic food before it gets to your local supermarket or restaurant must be certified, too. Look for the following seal as your way of knowing that the produce is organic.

> One of the criteria I use for shopping at a particular store is the quality of its produce. How fresh is it? How well is it displayed? What selections does it offer? My eyes enjoy the veritable kaleidoscope of colors, shapes, and textures as I walk through the aisles. Talk about "eye candy."

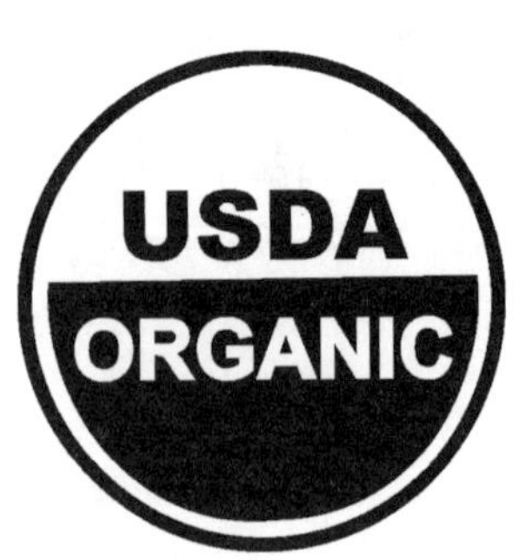

Certification seal for organically grown produce.

Are you the kind of shopper who heads for the more usual choices—like apples, bananas, and lettuce—without even glancing at some of the more unusual produce? When you see something that's unfamiliar, do you ever stop and ask the grocer what it is, what it tastes like, and how to prepare it? Many produce departments will give you a sample of something upon request. So it doesn't cost you a thing to explore.

By not eating a variety of fruits and vegetables, you may be missing the nutrition that a full range of choices can provide. For example, eating only bananas as your fruit means you may be getting a good supply of potassium, but you may be missing such vitamins as C and A found in oranges and apricots, respectively. I appreciate that our parents helped create many of our habits when we were young. What your parents ate, you ate. However, back when we were kids there were far fewer choices available than what you find today. Even if you could find some exotic fruit or vegetable back then, the price was prohibitive. Now, for example, you can get papaya from Hawaii and pay the same price on the mainland as you do on the islands.

If you were lost in the jungle and ran out of the food you had brought with you, would you pick fruit from the trees—even if that fruit was something you hadn't tried before? I know that survival makes people do things they might not ordinarily do, but it does show you that you could try something new.

I've heard people complain about the work involved in cleaning and cutting up vegetables. That would be a plausible excuse, except for the fact that grocery stores sell fresh, cut-up, and already cleaned vegetables in packages. You can even find cut-up fruit in the produce department. Next excuse! And even if you can't find them raw in the produce section, the frozen food aisle has plenty of cut-up varieties from plain string beans to fancy mixed vegetable combinations to melon pieces and berries.

Okay, is it the lack of ideas on how to prepare them? Most vegetables are good raw. If you don't enjoy them straight, you can serve them with some low-fat or fat-free salad dressings as a dip. Steaming vegetables and seasoning with some low-fat margarine and herbs can make them more interesting. I love grilled vegetables drizzled with a little olive oil. Add some to stews and casseroles. Soups are always a great way to include vegetables in your meal. How about Campbell's V-8 juice, where you get a variety of vegetables in one serving? Here's a piece of trivia for you: In 1948, former U.S. president Ronald Reagan, then an actor, served as the spokesman for V-8 juice. And do you remember back in the 1960s, where some of our vegetables came from? Answer: "From the valley of the jolly (ho, ho, ho) Green Giant."

The I-Don't-Like-Vegetables Soup

In a 4-quart saucepan, sauté one onion, chopped, in about 1 tablespoon olive oil until soft and limp. Add 4 cups vegetables. (You choose, but read Chapter 5 first.) I like to include carrots, broccoli, celery, and cauliflower. Add 1/2 cup split peas. Cover with 6 cups chicken broth (regular or unsalted). Add 1/4 to 1/2 teaspoon your favorite herbs (for example, *bouquet garni*), and bring to a boil. Turn the flame down and simmer for about 30 minutes or until vegetables are tender and split peas are softened. Allow the soup to cool slightly, and then purée in a blender in small batches. (Do not overfill. If you have a "pulse" switch on your blender, use it for a second or two to avoid having soup squirt out the lid. Then purée.) Season with salt and pepper to taste. Serve with a dollop (about 1 tablespoon) low-fat or nonfat plain yogurt. Tossing a couple croutons on the top can be a fun addition. *Note:* To make a complete meal in a bowl, add some cut-up cooked chicken or cooked fish to the soup as you serve it.

Tips for Eating More Vegetables and Fruits Every Day

To get you started on including more fruits and vegetables in your day, give some of these tips a try:

- Add strips of green or red bell pepper, carrot slices or grated carrots, sliced cucumber, broccoli florets, and shredded cabbage to give your salad, pasta, or potato salad color and crunch.
- Wake up your taste buds in the morning with a bowl of cereal topped with some sliced bananas, strawberries, blueberries, or raisins.
- Grill skewers of zucchini, onions, eggplant, cherry tomatoes, pineapple chunks, peaches or nectarines, and enjoy a taste treat.
- Give a sweet flavor to your coleslaw, tuna, or chicken by adding pineapple chunks, dates, chopped apple, raisins, or currants.
- The microwave is the most nutrient-friendly way to cook vegetables because it retains more nutrients than boiling.

- Think in terms of color and texture combinations—grapes with bananas; strawberries with rhubarb; various colored melons cut into balls with a melon ball cutter; medley of broccoli, cauliflower, yellow squash, and green peas.
- Fruits and vegetables can be added as a topper on almost anything you eat—pizza, yogurt, and sandwiches.
- When thirsty and on the go, take along 100 percent fruit juices or vegetable juices in easy-to-tote boxes or cans.
- Try store-bought cut-up vegetables and fruits for convenient snacks. Keep them handy and right up front in your refrigerator.
- Smoothies made in the blender are a great way to enjoy more fruits. Purée your choice of cut-up fruits with a little fruit juice and crushed ice. Want something richer? Add some nonfat fruit-flavored or vanilla-flavored yogurt.
- Add fruit juice to your salad dressing.
- Mother Nature provides fruits and vegetables in easy-to-carry packages that don't require peeling and chopping. Try baby carrots, grapes, cherry tomatoes, or broccoli florets.
- A healthier alternative to candy is dried fruit, such as dates, dried figs, prunes, raisins, dried apricots and apples. Just don't eat too much, because they're higher in calories per serving than their fresh counterparts.
- For a summer treat, make Popsicles of 100 percent fruit or vegetable juice. You could also make them in ice cube trays. Try adding the cubes to juice to avoid watering down your drink.
- Salsa made with tomatoes, mangoes, pineapple, cilantro, sweet onions, and lime juice provides a tasty low-fat dip for your low-fat chips.
- Be creative and adventurous—mix a variety of 100 percent fruit juices and see what flavor you get. Garnish with a mint sprig.

chapter 5

The Color System for Eating

Some things you have to do every day. Eating seven apples on Saturday night instead of one a day just isn't going to get the job done.

—Jim Rohn

The way I think about the color system for eating is the way I believe an artist thinks about the color palette for painting. Very few artists limit themselves to one color in a picture. How boring. The same holds true for the way we should color our diet. Although there are many variations of any particular color (for example, red and reddish purple), we can group fruits and vegetables into a palette of six basic colors: red, orange, yellow, green, white, and purple. Each of these color groups possesses its own profile of phytochemicals that makes it special. Yet there's much overlap among groups, not only in the phytochemicals they contain, but also in their vitamin and mineral content.

A Rainbow of Colors

Look at the Fruit and Vegetable Rainbow that follows. Notice that there are two green bands, Green 1 and Green 2. That's because the profile for the fruits and vegetables in each of those two bands is unique. Therefore, consider selecting from each group when you choose a "green" fruit or vegetable. Green 1 gives you sulforaphane, isothiocyanate, and indoles. Green 2 contains lutein and zeaxanthin. To see why these phytochemicals are so important to your health, there's a discussion at the end of the chapter.

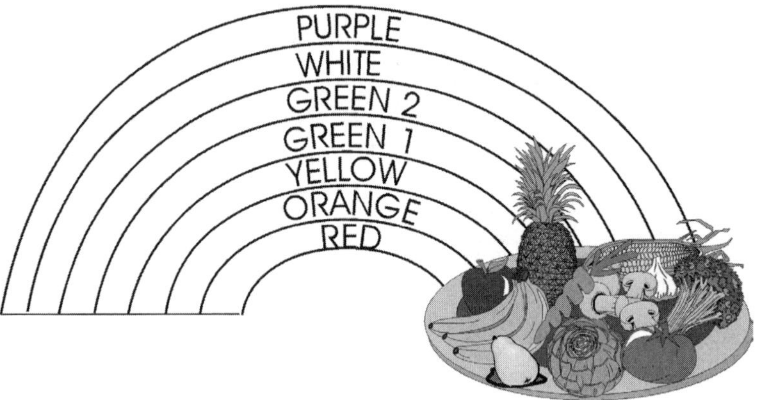

Fruit and Vegetable Rainbow.

The table that follows should help you with your selection of fruits and vegetables. By the end of the day, you should have eaten *at least* two colors of fruits and three colors of vegetables. If you're a sharp reader, you've probably realized that those numbers of servings represent the minimum numbers recommended on the Food Guide Pyramid and the 5-a-Day Program. You'll find how easy it is to get a variety of foods in your day by thinking in terms of colors.

For even more variety and nutrition, introduce a new color each day, allowing it to replace one that you had the day before. For example, today I'm having a banana and an orange for my two fruits. That takes care of the white and orange colors. (I know that a banana peel is yellow, but because we don't eat the peel, it's the color of the fruit itself that counts. On the other hand, a red apple is usually eaten with the skin, and it's the phytochemicals in the skin that make it part of the "red" group.) For my vegetables today, I'll select carrots, eggplant, and broccoli, satisfying the colors orange, purple, and green. By the way, you can have the same colors from the fruit group as you're having from the vegetable group. You can even select two different fruits or two different vegetables from the same color group if you want. With the choices I've made, I've gotten a good helping of potassium, vitamin C, beta-carotenes, sulforaphane, isothion-cyanate, and indoles. Tomorrow, I'll swap the orange for a piece of papaya, and the string beans for spinach. By doing that, I'm still getting a good supply of all the same nutrients, but have now added some vitamin A, lutein, and zeaxanthin.

> It's how your nutrition adds up for the week that matters. No one day necessarily has to contain every nutrient. If you've eaten a wide variety of foods throughout the week, you'll probably get a complete supply of the nutrients your body needs.

I also like to consider what colors I'll include on my plate just to make it more attractive. Having, for example, turkey, mashed potatoes, and cauliflower would make a pretty boring-looking plate. Everything looks white. On the other hand, if instead of the cauliflower, I had a mixed medley of broccoli, carrots, and red bell peppers, I would spiff up my plate. Don't ever forget that part of the pleasure in eating is the eye appeal of what you're eating. Watch a food program on television and you'll see what I mean. Presentation is half the fun of cooking.

Selecting Fruits and Vegetables by Color

Color	Fruits	Vegetables
Red	Pink grapefruit	Radish
	Pink guava	Red bell peppers
	Red apple	Tomato
	Red pear	Tomato juice
	Rhubarb	
	Strawberries	
	Watermelon	

continues

Selecting Fruits and Vegetables by Color *(continued)*

Color	Fruits	Vegetables
Orange	Apricot	Acorn squash
	Cantaloupe	Carrot juice
	Mango	Carrots
	Nectarine	Orange bell peppers
	Orange	Pumpkin
	Papaya	Sweet potato
	Peach	Winter squash
	Tangerine	Yam
Yellow	Grapefruit	Corn
	Lemon	Yellow bell peppers
	Pineapple	Yellow squash
Green 1		Bok choy
		Broccoli
		Brussels sprouts
		Cabbage
		Chinese cabbage
		Kale
Green 2	Green apple	Avocado
	Green grapes	Chicory
	Green pear	Collard greens
	Honeydew melon	Cucumber
		Green beans
		Green peas
		Leaf lettuce
		Mustard greens
		Romaine lettuce
		Spinach
		Swiss chard
		Turnip greens
		Zucchini

Color	Fruits	Vegetables
White	Banana	Cauliflower
		Celery
		Endive
		Garlic
		Onion
Purple	Blackberries	Beets
	Blueberries	Eggplant
	Cherries	Red cabbage
	Cranberries	
	Cranberry juice	
	Figs	
	Grape juice	
	Plum	
	Plums	
	Prunes	
	Red grapes	
	Red wine	

Now You're Cooking

The way you cook your vegetables will affect how much of these valuable phytochemicals are left in the food for you to eat. Microwaving your vegetables preserves the most vitamins, whereas boiling them removes the most. Broiling, grilling, and roasting are also good ways of cooking. Fortunately, the minerals in vegetables remain intact during cooking. What's interesting is that, in some cases, cooking releases the phytochemicals to make them more available to your body. This is true of *lycopene* in tomatoes and *beta-carotene* in carrots. That's not to say that you can't eat them raw, because they still are healthy choices. On the other hand, *sulforaphane* that's found in broccoli and cauliflower is more bio-available when these vegetables are eaten raw. When you consider the sulfur smell of overcooked broccoli and cauliflower, you can imagine that many of the phytochemicals are lost in the cooking process. Our grandparents and even some of our parents probably cooked their vegetables in baking soda as a way of preserving their color. What they didn't know, though, was that baking soda can destroy the vitamin C content of vegetables.

Understanding All Those Scientific Terms

There has been, and will continue to be, a great deal of research on phytochemicals. When you and I were younger, people talked in terms of the food itself. Now, with modern technology, scientists talk more about what the food contains. What's even more fascinating is how the body deals with these nutrients.

The following list should help familiarize you with terms you'll be hearing more and more about in the news. Please don't panic—there won't be a test at the end of the chapter to see what you can remember. Just read this list for a basic understanding of why these phytochemicals are important. Be thankful that Mother Nature has given us so much protection in the foods we eat (that is, if you eat your fruits and vegetables!).

- **Anthocyanins** contribute the red and reddish-purple color to grapes, grape juice, red wine, red cabbage, eggplant, and radishes. As one of the flavonoids, they can protect against heart disease and cancer.
- **Antioxidants** have the potential for preventing cancer, heart disease, and even the damages caused by old age. (As baby boomers, anything we can do to ward off the effects of getting older is, in my opinion, well worth trying. Also, we're still young enough to *prevent* these diseases, rather than having to *treat* them.) Many of the names of the antioxidants sound really scientific (such as *resveratrol* and *carotenoids*). It almost makes you think that you'd have to go to a chemist to have some cooked up in a brew or go to your local nutrition supplement store to get them in a pill. Let me save you the money and the trip. Just eat your fruits and vegetables.

  So how do antioxidants work? We can't live without oxygen. Yet it seems ironic that oxygen, in certain forms, can be destructive to our body. The cellular activity that keeps us alive can produce damaging by-products known as "free radicals." (When I said free radicals, did you think I was referring to the rebels during the free-speech movement in the 1960s?!) External elements can also create free radicals in the body—elements such as cigarette smoke (firsthand and secondhand), alcohol, x-rays, ultraviolet light, and other pollutants. Free radicals are unstable oxygen molecules that move around in the body looking for something that will make them more stable. Antioxidants made in the body and those supplied from food can stabilize free radicals—an obvious benefit. Because there are lots of free radicals formed or entering your body every day, you need a good supply of antioxidants onboard. Limiting your exposure to external sources of free radicals will greatly help.

Not all free radicals exist for evil purposes. Sometimes they defend the body against invaders. But when free radicals attack healthy cells, they can cause problems such as cancer or heart disease. They can even go after and tamper with DNA, our body's blueprint for making new cells. Obviously, that's the last thing we want happening.

Each antioxidant does a different job. That's why it's so important to eat a variety of fruits and vegetables. No single fruit or vegetable has all we need to wage a war against free radicals. For those of you thinking, "I'll just pop a pill and then I won't have to eat the fruits and vegetables," think again. Research is showing that it may be the combination of some or all of the other nutrients in fruits and vegetables working together that creates the beneficial effect. We need to begin thinking more in terms of the "whole" rather than the parts; that the sum of what we eat is greater than each individual food, and that each food is greater than its individual nutrients.

- **Carotenoids** give such foods as carrots, yams, and apricots their orange color. Carotenoids are another form of antioxidant, with beta-carotene having gotten most of the attention until lately. Lutein and lycopene are in the spotlight for their ability to fight against cataracts and prostate cancer. With many hundreds of carotenoids in the fruits and vegetables we eat, it will be a long time before all of them are identified.

- **Ellagic acid** is found in blackberries, raspberries, cranberries, strawberries, grapes, and walnuts, and is thought to have anticancer properties that deactivate carcinogens (cancer-causing compounds).
- **Flavonoids** in fruits, vegetables, nuts, and grains act as powerful antioxidants. They increase vitamin C activity, protect the bad variety of cholesterol (LDL cholesterol) from being oxidized (which can lead to plaque formation and heart disease), and inhibit platelets from clumping together. They can also help protect against inflammation and tumor growth. *Quercetin* is one of the major flavonoids that you'll find in broccoli, kale, onions, grapes, green beans, apples, and cereals. It may be involved in the "French Paradox"—the finding that even though French people eat a high-fat diet, their incidence of coronary artery disease is low. The value of quercetin, which is found in grape skins, is related to lipid (fat) regulation and antithrombotic (anticlotting) capabilities. Of course, while the French enjoy their wine, which may be part of the reason for the French Paradox, they also eat more fruits and vegetables than we do. The sulfides in onions and garlic may be involved in inhibiting the growth of bacteria that could lead to stomach cancer. They can lower blood pressure and influence the immune system. Have some tea, especially green tea, and you'll be getting a good dose of *catechins*.
- **Isoflavones** are found mainly in soybeans and are credited with reducing some heart disease problems, preventing some unpleasant side effects of menopause (such as bone loss and hot flashes) by acting as phytoestrogens, and may decrease the risk of prostate, breast, and other cancers. Isoflavones are chemically very similar to the male hormone testosterone and the female hormone estrogen. Because of that, they're attracted to sites in the body to which these hormones normally bind and may therefore interfere with the hormone's involvement in the development of cancer.

(However, some women who have had breast cancer are advised to minimize their intake of soy products due to this subtle estrogen effect of the soy isoflavones. Consult with your doctor to be certain whether you should include soy in your diet.) Some other compounds that make soybeans so powerful in their fight against cancer are *genistein, daidzein,* and *saponins.* With names like that, they sound like they must be good for you.

- **Lutein** and **zeaxanthin** are found in spinach, kale, and turnip greens, and may help reduce the risk of cancer.
- **Lycopene** is another form of antioxidant, found in fruits and vegetables that are red or pink in color such as tomatoes, red bell peppers, pink guava, and pink grapefruit. There is strong evidence linking a decreased risk of prostate cancer in men who eat foods high in lycopene. To make the lycopene from tomatoes more available to the body, it's best to eat cooked tomatoes (for example, stewed tomatoes and tomato sauces).
- **Resveratrol** is a compound that may lower the risk of cancer and heart disease. A good source is grapes and grape juice, with red grapes having greater amounts than green grapes. If you're not a wine drinker, you don't have to start. Other phytochemicals will protect you.
- **Sulforaphane** in cruciferous vegetables such as broccoli, cauliflower, Brussels sprouts, kale, cabbage, and bok choy stimulates the body to produce cancer-fighting proteins.

chapter 6

Mares Eat Oats, and So Should You

"Seven out of ten people suffer from hemorrhoids."
Does this mean that the other three enjoy it?
—Sal Davino

Left to their own devices, animals will eat naturally and very well, as long as food is available. Cows go for the greener grass (which always seems to be on the other side of the fence). Horses love oats, and some pigs relish truffles (talk about expensive dining!). Then why is it that humans, who are supposed to be the smartest in the brains department, sometimes eat the least healthy foods?

When the starving people of France were revolting against the aristocracy, Marie Antoinette responded, "Let them eat cake." That goes to show you how much she knew about good nutrition. (Actually, it shows you how insensitive the aristocracy was to the needs of their people. But that discussion is best left for another book.) At that time in France, only the very rich could afford refined flour and sugar. The peasants had to eat whole grains. Had the people not lacked food, or lived in such squalid conditions, they might have been able to live to an old age. Eating whole grains was healthier for them than the refined flour and sugar eaten by the aristocracy.

I don't know about you, but I can never get the lyrics straight for that song "Mares Eat Oats." If you're curious, here's how it sounds, followed by the "real" words:

Mairzy doats
And dozy doats
And liddle lamzy divey.
A kiddley divey too,
Wouldn't you?

Mare's eat oats,
And does eat oats,
And little lambs eat ivy.
A kid'll eat ivy, too.
Wouldn't a ewe?

Food Label Claim Allowed by the FDA

Diets low in saturated fat and cholesterol and high in fiber are associated with a reduced risk of certain cancers, diabetes, digestive disorders, and heart disease.

Somehow, we haven't yet learned the lesson. We still have a love affair with refined flour and sugar. Remember, we grew up with Wonder Bread, the ultimate white bread! But that was then, and this is now. It's time to act like an adult and take responsibility for eating what's best for you. The average American eats only about 11 grams of fiber a day, even though the recommendation for those of you boomers who are 50 years or younger is 38 grams per day if you're a man and 25 grams if you're a woman. For those boomers who are older than 50, 30 grams for men and 21 grams for women. The fact that the Food and Drug Administration (FDA) will now allow fiber claims to appear on a food label tells you how important a matter this is.

When we were growing up, the only time you heard about fiber was when your parents were suffering from constipation. You'd know about it when the box of bran cereal and prunes came home with the groceries. Maybe some parents who were a little more health-oriented bought whole-wheat bread. Today the choices are endless and far tastier.

A Little Bit of History

It was probably Dr. Denis Burkitt who brought the "fiber story" to the attention of the public. He was working with native Africans in Uganda and noticed that these people were not suffering from the typical diseases found in Western countries. They didn't seem to have the rate of colon cancer, diverticulosis (pouches formed in the wall of the colon that become infected), hemorrhoids, or varicose veins that was typical of Western cultures in the 1960s and 1970s. From observing what they ate, Burkitt concluded that the diet of these African people, being high in grains and plant foods and low in animal products, was protecting them from these diseases.

It's not that Burkitt was the first to appreciate the value of fiber. Even Hippocrates, the father of modern medicine, knew that whole grain was good for the bowels. Roman athletes even ate it, thinking it gave them strength. Yet the general population in the eighteenth and nineteenth centuries looked at whole-wheat bread and bran as something only for the poor.

With the introduction of modern sieve rolling mills in the late nineteenth century, white flour became more readily available and more economical than before. Now more people were eating refined flour. Back then, it wasn't known that by refining the flour, valuable vitamins such as thiamine and niacin were being removed. Cases of beriberi (due to thiamine deficiency) and pellagra (due to niacin deficiency) increased dramatically in the early twentieth century. When the reason for the deficiencies was discovered, the United States government made vitamin and mineral fortification of flour a requirement. Yet, how sad to remove something nutritional and have to add it back (and by the way, it never all does get put back), all for the sake of having white flour. Many of the valuable phytochemicals also are lost.

Americans have been suffering from indigestion for centuries. In the early 1800s, Sylvester Graham thought he had the answer. All that refined flour was doing the American population in. He recommended putting bran back into the diet. He created the "graham cracker," which was made from graham (whole-wheat) flour. I'm not sure how many of the graham crackers today are 100 percent whole wheat, but at least Graham was on the right track. However, Americans were too in love with their white bread to embrace Graham's approach. Fiber intake has continued to decline. Graham thought he had the solution to America's indigestion problems—eat more bran; today Americans try to find the remedy in antacids. What are they thinking?

Know Your Fibers

While all fibers are not the same, they do have one thing in common—they can't be totally broken down by human digestive enzymes and absorbed by the body. You might wonder why you should bother eating fiber when it never gets absorbed. Read on and find out why adding more fiber to your diet is a healthy thing to do.

There are two types of fiber—*insoluble* and *soluble*. The soluble and insoluble fibers serve many purposes, functioning differently in the gastrointestinal tract. Many foods contain both fibers.

The major function of **insoluble fiber** is to decrease the time food spends in the intestine. It used to be thought that potential cancer-causing compounds, called *carcinogens,* would get trapped in the fiber as it moved along the intestinal tract. These carcinogens would then have less opportunity to cause colon cancer. Studies are proving this not to be the case. But don't give up on insoluble fiber. By making the walls of your intestine work harder, it makes them stronger. Consider fiber as weight lifting for your intestines. Fiber increases bulk and helps to eliminate *constipation* (as long as you drink plenty of fluids with it), which makes for a healthier intestine. Eating fiber may also help with *obesity* because it can trap some of the fats in the food you eat, preventing them from being absorbed.

Soluble fiber is different from insoluble fiber in that it is able to make a gel. It draws water to itself. By doing so, the fiber helps make the stomach empty more slowly, which causes you to feel full longer and, hopefully, not overeat. Soluble fiber can also be good for people with *diabetes.* Their body cannot handle a great deal of sugar at one time. Because the stomach empties more slowly, soluble fiber promotes a slower absorption of sugar and conversion of carbohydrates to glucose. This gives the body a chance to maintain better control of the blood sugar level. Soluble fiber can also be very good for people with a cholesterol problem or *heart disease.* Dietary cholesterol becomes bound up in the gel, allowing less of it to be absorbed by the body. Oatmeal is an example of a healthy grain with soluble fiber that you should add to your diet, because it does a great job of trapping cholesterol.

You may hear terms such as *lignan, cellulose, hemicellulose,* and *pectin* used when people refer to fiber. Unless you really have a burning interest in the chemical makeup of fiber, I wouldn't worry about them. Just know that if you eat a balanced diet with plenty of fruits, vegetables, whole grains, and legumes, you'll do just fine. Look in Appendix A for a list of foods and their fiber content for help in making healthy selections.

> Good sources of soluble fiber: Fruits, vegetables, legumes, and oats
>
> Good sources of insoluble fiber: Whole-wheat and whole-grain products, especially wheat bran and brown rice, vegetables

Spotlight on Soy

Highlighting soy is not meant to make less of any of the other legumes. However, much research has been done to determine the benefits of soy, which seem to be many.

Any postmenopausal woman having hot flashes probably has heard, and maybe even thought, about taking soy supplements or adding soy to her diet. Because soy has a phytoestrogen-type activity, it can fake the body out in clever ways. By appearing to be an estrogen, it can bind to estrogen receptors in the breast, uterus, and ovaries, blocking real estrogen from getting there first. By so doing, there could be a decreased risk of hormone-sensitive *cancers* affecting these parts of the body. I say "could" because some health professionals are concerned that soy can act like estrogen, not just bind like estrogen. If you're at a high risk for breast cancer, limit your intake of soy products. Otherwise, it might be a good alternative to hormone replacement therapy. It is highly recommended that you consult your physician first. Men may also want to consider adding soy to their diet. Although the data are limited, the primary isoflavone in soybeans, *genistein,* seems to inhibit the growth of hormone-dependent and -independent prostate cancer cells.

Another benefit of soy's estrogenlike activity is on *bone* health. Many postmenopausal women take estrogen to protect against osteoporosis. Yet with hormone replacement therapy still being in question as a possible link with breast cancer, maybe eating soy protein would be the answer. Its isoflavones might have estrogenic effect on the bones by slowing bone turnover. Unless you select a soy milk that is fortified with calcium, don't look to it for your calcium intake for the day. Check the label for its calcium content.

Soy protein seems to have a cholesterol-lowering capability, according to some studies. Even the FDA in 1999 thought there was enough correlation to allow a health claim on soy protein's ability to reduce heart disease, as long as it was accompanied by a low-saturated-fat and low-cholesterol diet. The claim stated you would have to eat 25 grams of soy protein a day to reduce the risk of heart disease. There are those in the research field who think soy proteins are involved in reducing one's risk of cardiac heart disease by lowering levels of the bad LDL cholesterol, without disturbing the good HDL cholesterol levels. Some of soy's benefits are related to its antioxidant activity and effect on the dilation and constriction of the blood vessels. This, in turn, can affect blood pressure.

Just in its role as a fiber, soy can help delay emptying of the stomach and delay absorption of sugars, and so is beneficial to someone with diabetes. It may even lower one's risk for colon cancer. Because it contains oligosaccharides (sugars that our intestines can't break down), the bifidobacteria in the large intestine thrive. These, in turn, inhibit the growth of pathogenic bacteria by creating a more acidic environment.

After all this discussion, you may think soy is the wonder food of the twenty-first century. Although it has many health benefits, don't ignore other good sources of fiber for the job they can do.

If you check out the following table, you'll see how you might be able to eat 25 milligrams of soy protein a day with the foods listed.

Good Sources of Soy Protein

Source	Amount	Grams of Soy Protein
Soy protein isolate	4 tablespoons	23
Dry soy protein	4 tablespoons	13 to 23
Tempeh (fermented soy cake)	4 ounces	17
Tofu	4 ounces	13

Source	Amount	Grams of Soy Protein
Baked soy nuts	1/4 cup	12
Edamame (raw green beans)	3 ounces	10
Soy milk	1 cup	4 to 8

Note: Tofu can also be a fairly good source of calcium, depending on its preparation. Look on the label for its ingredients and see if calcium chloride or calcium sulfate are listed. These are the coagulants used to thicken soy milk into the block of tofu. Many brands of soy milk are fortified with calcium.

Because tofu is fairly bland, it can be added to many foods and not change the flavor dramatically. For example, use tofu in casseroles, stir-fries, or brown it like a piece of meat. Add it to soup, and then purée the soup for a creamy finish. Soy milk works in many recipes that call for regular milk.

Many boomers have gone vegetarian, realizing that it takes far less resources to grow the food that feeds people a vegetarian diet than a meat-based diet. In many ways, it does seem like the "responsible" thing to do. They appreciate that soy is a good alternative to meat as their protein source.

Making Friends with Fiber

If you haven't been including a lot of fiber in your diet up to this point, then let me suggest you make friends with it on a gradual basis. Add a few extra grams every 2 or 3 days until you reach the goal of 20 to 35 grams per day. Make sure you drink plenty of fluids, at least eight glasses per day. Remember that fiber absorbs water. If you forget the fluids, you're going to have one hard rock in your intestines.

If beans cause you (or others!) discomfort because of gas, try products such as Beano or Say Yes To Beans. Let me share with you why the body gets gassy after you eat beans. (There are those who will call it "flatulence," so it doesn't sound so crude a subject to talk about.) There is a sugar in beans called *raffinose.* The body doesn't have an enzyme in the small intestine that can break down the sugar. So the sugar passes into your large intestine intact. However, the bacteria there find it a great feast and are more than happy to break it down. As they do, they produce gas as a by-product. When you use such products as Beano or Say Yes To Beans, the enzymes in these products help break the sugar down in the small intestine, providing less for the bacteria to feed on and less gas by-products.

You may be tempted to rely on fiber supplements rather than get fiber from your food. If you're eating a balanced diet, you should be getting plenty of fiber, and at least it will be both soluble and insoluble. Besides, why pay extra for a fiber supplement, when that money could go to the food you eat? Just learn to choose wisely. A bowl of bran cereal each morning, a dish of beans, and a healthy helping of fruits and vegetables each day may be all you need. If you still feel you want to take a supplement, go for the bulk-forming ones, such as psyllium, flaxseed, pectin, or guar gum, being sure to drink plenty of fluids with them. Just keep in mind that most researchers believe that it's the combination of insoluble and soluble fibers found in food that is most protective of your intestines.

Please try not to rely on laxatives to keep everything moving. The intestines can get lazy and very dependent on them. In the old days, people used to use mineral oil as a laxative. Fat-soluble vitamins got trapped in the mineral oil and never were absorbed. People then became deficient in such vitamins as A and D.

Cooking Beans

Soak the beans in water overnight, if possible. If you don't have the time, then put them in a pot, cover with water, and bring the water to a boil. Turn off the heat and let stand for an hour. Drain the water and then add more water to cover. Bring the pot back to a boil and simmer until tender. Throwing off the first water removes some of the substances that can cause you gas.

Fiber Tips

Read labels. Unless a food doesn't have any fiber, the label should tell you how many grams there are in a serving. Go for products that have a fiber %DV (Daily Value) of 20. It means you're getting a high source, at least 5 grams. Ignore such statements as "made with wheat" or "made with natural whole grain" on the front of food packages and go directly to the list of ingredients. If the first ingredient is "whole wheat" or "whole grain," you've got a good source of fiber. If it says "enriched wheat," that doesn't mean it's whole grain—just that some of the nutrients were put back into the flour. A product made with oats isn't going to say "whole oats," because oats aren't refined like flour. So as long as the first ingredient in the list is oats, that's the largest contributor to the ingredients.

Whenever possible, eat whole-grain products. Make your bread and your pasta whole wheat. Eat brown rice instead of white rice. Add wheat germ to your bowl of cereal. Be adventurous and try products like couscous and kasha.

Raw vegetables have more fiber than cooked vegetables, because the cooking process can break down some of the fiber. If you do cook your veggies, do them in the microwave oven until just crisp and tender. The microwave does a better job of preserving the fiber than boiling them, and less of the nutrients are lost. Raw vegetables are a great snack. Have them cut up and handy in the refrigerator.

If you clean your vegetables and fruits really well, eat them with their skins. There's a lot of soluble fiber in the skins. Because juice contains less fiber, opt for whole vegetables and fruits when you can. As an example, 1 medium orange has about 3 grams fiber, whereas 4 ounces orange juice has a mere ½ gram fiber.

Pop some cooked beans and legumes in your soups, stews, pasta dishes, and casseroles. They even go well on a salad.

Be adventurous and try some of these exciting grains in such products as cereals, breads, and pastas: amaranth, kasha (buckwheat groats), quinoa, spelt, and triticale.

Even though dried fruit is higher in calories than fresh fruit, it does have a good amount of fiber. Occasionally opt for dried fruit as a snack, treat, or dessert. Dried plums are a good source of both insoluble and soluble fibers. (I think the growers of these fruits decided to change the name from prunes to dried plums because none of us baby boomers wanted to eat the fruit our grandparents and parents ate when they were constipated.)

Check Appendix A for a sample day's menu showing how you can increase your fiber.

Picks for Your Fiber Fix

Food	Grams of Fiber
Whole-grain products	2 to 3 grams
Dry beans, lentils, peas	6 to 8 grams
Fruits and vegetables	2 to 3 grams
Nuts and seeds	2 to 3 grams

chapter 7

Fat Isn't a Four-Letter Word

As for butter versus margarine, I trust cows more than chemists.

—Joan Gussow

It's amazing how many people suffer from fat phobia. The media have helped promote the fear by making people feel that eating fat will surely make them fat. The food manufacturers are only too happy to provide the plethora of fat-free and low-fat products that consumers are more than willing to buy every year. Yet, in their attempt to avoid fat, people unknowingly and naïvely are eating more calories and more sugar. Many fat-free and low-fat products have as many calories as their full-fat counterparts, because sugar is added to make them taste good. With a mind-set that the food is fat-free, people eat without restriction, ignoring the fact that these products are not calorie-free.

Let's get one thing straight. All of us need some fat in our diet. There are certain fatty acids the human body can't make—they can only be supplied from what we eat. Dietary fat also helps transport fat-soluble nutrients like vitamins A, D, E, and K, as well as beta-carotene. From a pleasure point of view, fat gives food flavor. It also helps with satiety (a feeling of fullness). The fact that Americans are still eating too much fat doesn't mean you need to give it all up. However, being more selective would be healthful.

When we were growing up, few people talked about "fatty acids." They merely said something was either high in fat or not. Research has now shown that we need to understand what the three different fatty acids are—saturated, polyunsaturated, and monounsaturated—and what foods they're found in (see the following figure).

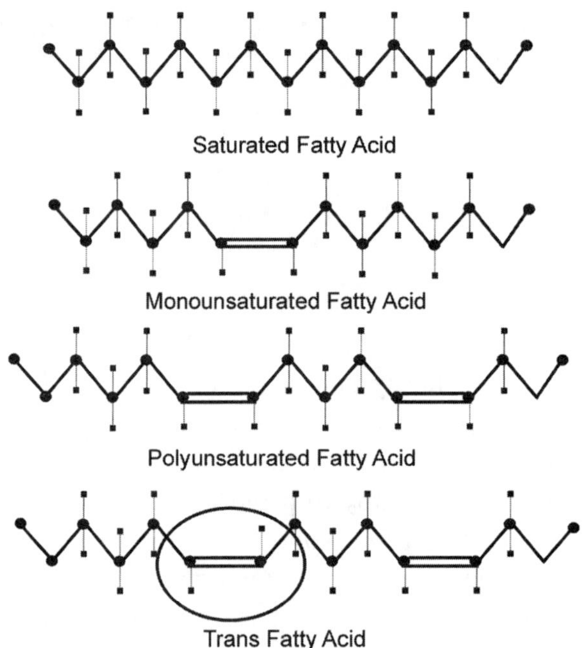

The little squares on the ends of the thin lines represent hydrogen atoms. The little circles at the peak of each sawtooth represent carbon atoms. The double lines represent double bonds.

Saturated fatty acids are the building blocks of saturated fats. They're the ones to worry about. Too much of these and you increase your risk for heart disease by potentially elevating the "bad" LDL cholesterol in your blood. At the same time, these fats decrease the "good" HDL cholesterol. That's not a good formula for heart health. The

American Heart Association recommends that no more than 10 percent of calories come from saturated fat. If you already have heart disease, that percentage should be dropped to less than 7 percent. You find saturated fats in abundance in meats, high-fat dairy products (cheeses, ice cream, butter), and in some tropical oils (coconut oil, palm oil, palm kernel oil). A way to recognize a saturated fat is that it's solid at room temperature. From the preceding figure, notice that there are no double lines on the saturated fat. That means it's literally saturated with hydrogen atoms. The fatty acid can't take on any more.

Monounsaturated fatty acids are found in olive, canola, peanut, and other nut oils. They tend to beneficially raise the level of the good HDL cholesterol without also raising the level of bad LDL cholesterol, as long as the rest of your diet is low in saturated fats and calories. The Mediterranean diet is high in monounsaturated fats and low in saturated fats. People in Mediterranean countries eat very little meat, and get a good deal of monounsaturated fat from olive oil. Looking at the diagram, you can see how there's one set of double lines or bonds. That means that two more hydrogen atoms can be added to the fatty acid. So this fat isn't saturated.

> Extra-virgin olive oil is the oil that comes from the first cold pressing of the olives, using no heat or chemicals. It's rich in flavor and antioxidants. It costs more than virgin olive oil or olive oil, the latter being extracted using chemicals. An olive oil with less acid, such as extra-virgin olive oil, will have a better flavor.

Polyunsaturated fatty acids are like monounsaturated fatty acids, but have more than one double bond. They, too, help decrease LDL cholesterol. With numerous double bonds, they have plenty of spaces to take on more hydrogen atoms if they need to. You'll hear references to *omega-3 fatty acids* and *omega-6 fatty acids,* both in this book and in the news. Two fatty acids, *alpha-linolenic* and *linoleic,* from these families of fatty acids are considered "essential" because your body can't make them. That means you have to get them from your diet.

You'll find omega-3s in deep cold-water fatty fish (for example, salmon, tuna, sardines, halibut, and herring), and, more specifically, the alpha-linolenic acid in canola, soybean, flaxseed, and walnut oils. Some foods that are rich in omegas-6s and linoleic acid are vegetable oils (such as corn, safflower, sunflower, and soybean) and nuts and seeds. The typical American diet is much higher in omega-6 fatty acids than omega-3s. That's why health professionals are now recommending that we eat at least two servings of fish per week. It'll increase our intake of two particular omega-3 fatty acids—*docosahexaenoic acid* (DHA) and *eicosapentaenoic acid* (EPA). The omega fatty acids can do many good things for the body:

- Help regulate blood pressure and heart rate
- Make your blood less sticky, so it's not as likely to form clots
- Support your immune response
- Protect against arthritis and stroke

> You may be wondering what the number after the word omega means. When you count the number of carbon atoms from one end of the fatty acid, it's where you'll find the first double bond. So for example, look at the polyunsaturated fatty acid in the preceding figure. From the left side, count each of the circles until you reach the sixth circle. That's where the double bond starts. That's an omega-6 fatty acid. The same process would be true for the omega-3 fatty acid, except the double bond would start at the third carbon atom.

The fat that's been getting a great deal of attention lately is the *trans fatty acid.* It acts like a saturated fat, increasing LDL cholesterol and lowering HDL cholesterol, an unhealthy combination. When you look at the diagram in the preceding figure, you may wonder why that's true—it has some double bonds. Let me explain by sharing with you how trans fatty acids come about. A major contributor of trans fatty acids in the diet is margarine, along with baked and fried foods. These foods contain *hydrogenated* or *partially hydrogenated* oils. (Check food ingredient labels to see.) The process of hydrogenating oil forces hydrogen atoms onto some of the double bonds, saturating them (removing the double bond). It also changes the placement of the hydrogen atoms around some of the double bonds. If you look at the diagram of the trans fatty acid, you can see that the hydrogen atoms are no longer on the same side of the double bond as they were in the polyunsaturated fatty acid. One has flipped. This could be even more detrimental to the body than saturated fat if you get too much of it.

The reason for hydrogenation is to make a liquid oil, such as corn oil or safflower oil, into something more solid at room temperature. (It's definitely much easier for spreading on toast!) It also gives fat a longer shelf life, and improves the texture of some foods. The healthier margarines will have liquid oil listed first in the ingredients and, therefore, have less trans fatty acids than stick margarine. The "light" margarines are even better because water replaces some of the fat. Again, look at the consistency of the product as your guide. The harder it is, the more trans fatty acids or saturated fats it contains. You can now buy margarines that are made without trans fats. In addition, the government will soon be requiring manufacturers to state on the label the amount of trans fatty acids in a food. Many people wonder: If margarine has these unhealthy trans fatty acids, shouldn't I just go back to eating butter? The answer is no, because butter is still mostly saturated fat, which, as I said earlier, is not a heart-healthy fat. You can't avoid eating some trans fatty acids, because they do occur naturally in some foods. However, the level in those foods is quite low compared to processed foods, which Americans consume in great quantity.

No food contains purely one fatty acid—all foods contain a combination. It's a matter of which one predominates. Check out Appendix B to see which fats contain the highest amount of saturated fatty acids, monounsaturated fatty acids, and polyunsaturated fatty acids. Make your selection accordingly, keeping in mind the benefits and the downside of the particular fatty acid.

A discussion of fat would not be complete without mentioning cholesterol. I just want to be sure that you don't confuse dietary cholesterol with blood cholesterol. There is no good or bad cholesterol in food. It only becomes good (HDL cholesterol) or bad (LDL cholesterol) in your body. The only place you'll find dietary cholesterol is in animal products (for example, in meat, poultry, dairy products, seafood, and eggs). Studies have shown that dietary cholesterol causes less increase in blood cholesterol than saturated fats do. That's why it's so important to watch how much saturated fat you're getting in your diet. Many people avoid shellfish because it's fairly high in cholesterol; yet it's low in saturated fats. So there's no reason you can't enjoy it occasionally. Just keep in mind the American Heart Association's recommendation of eating less than 300 milligrams of dietary cholesterol per day, or less than 200 milligrams if you have heart disease. Read your food labels to find out how much is in the food you're eating.

Setting a Good Example

The dairy industry has done a great job of providing consumers with low-fat and nonfat milk products. In the mid 1950s, people were beginning to switch from whole milk to low-fat milk. For some, the changeover was difficult. By the 1970s, though, with many more Americans concerned about eating too many fatty foods, sales of low-fat milk increased dramatically. Now almost all dairy products can be purchased in a low-fat or nonfat version.

Cheeses have also been made into lower-fat versions, some more successfully than others. As long as you don't want to melt them, the low-fat cheeses are fine. If you do choose a full-fat cheese, just eat less of it. Here's another suggestion. If you select a stronger-flavored cheese, you won't need to eat as much to receive flavor satisfaction. It's up to you how you want to spend your fat allowance.

> Do you remember the glass milk bottles sold in grocery stores or delivered to your door? When it was found that the light destroyed the riboflavin in the milk, the glass bottles were replaced with opaque containers.

One dairy product that can't be made into a lower-fat version is butter. We eat less butter now than we did when we were growing up. However, there was a time during World War II, when butter became so expensive and unavailable that an interest in margarine was rekindled. Margarine isn't anything new. It has existed for years. In fact, in 1870, a Frenchman developed it in response to a request by Emperor Louis Napoleon III to create a satisfactory replacement for butter. It would have taken off in the United States, except for protests from the dairy industry, which culminated in the Margarine Act of 1886. The act imposed a tax on margarine and required expensive licensing for the manufacture of margarine.

To further restrict margarine from replacing butter, the states instituted color laws. Margarine manufacturers weren't allowed to add any color to their product—that was to make sure it didn't look like butter. To get around that, manufacturers sold the white margarine in a sealed plastic bag that contained a capsule of color.

As baby boomers, we were too young to appreciate margarine in its infancy. My husband, who was born slightly before the baby boomer era, remembers his mother giving him the job of breaking the capsule and slowly kneading the food dye into the white vegetable shortening "oleo," until it was thoroughly colored. This could not have sat well with famous chefs like Julia Child. Today, margarines command a lot of shelf space in the market and, understandably so, when you appreciate the amount of saturated fat in butter. However, I have to agree with Julia Child when she says there are times when only butter will do. I just count it toward my saturated fat allowance for the day.

What's It Worth?

When you see a stick of butter, a piece of lard, or a bottle of oil, you know you're getting 100 percent fat. But what about those foods that have hidden fat? Those are the ones that will most likely get you into trouble. With fat having 9 calories per gram, compared to the 4 calories that a gram of protein or carbohydrate has, you're talking about an energy-dense nutrient.

In Appendix C you'll find two tables that should give you a very visual idea of just how much fat you're getting with some of the foods you might be eating. The tables show how many teaspoons of fat are in each of the foods. If you want to figure out how many teaspoons of fat are in something you're eating, look at the food label and divide the grams of Total Fat by five. When you eat at a fast-food restaurant, ask for their Nutrition Facts brochure, so you can figure out the number of teaspoons of fat in something you plan to eat (or just ate!). You might just change your mind.

You need to decide what it's worth to you to eat a particular food, based on how much fat it contains. To do that, it would be helpful to know how many teaspoons of fat you can have per day. In Chapter 16, you'll find out how many calories are right for you. When you know that number, come back here to see what that means in terms of how much fat you can have (based on 30 percent of total calories). This isn't just added fat I'm talking about. It's all the fat, both what you see and what you can't see.

Calories	Grams Total Fat	Teaspoons Total Fat	Grams Saturated Fat	Teaspoons Saturated Fat
1,200	40	8	13	2⅔
1,500	50	10	17	3⅓
1,800	60	12	20	4
2,100	70	14	23	4⅔
2,400	80	16	27	5⅓

Let's say that you're supposed to be eating 1,800 calories per day. For lunch, you decide to have the Burger King Original Double Whopper with Cheese. That Double Whopper is going to turn out to be a big whoops! It's got 14 teaspoons of fat, and you're only allowed 12 *for the day*. Too much! And, by the way, you have other meals to eat, which are likely to have some fat in them. How did you plan to fit those in?

Faux Fat

In our attempts to have it all, Procter & Gamble came up with what they thought was the answer—olestra. Olestra, a fat substitute sold under the trade name, Olean, has the mouth feel of fat without the calories of fat. It is such a big molecule that the body can't absorb it. So it just travels on through the digestive tract and out. This seemed like a dream come true. Food that spent a moment on our lips wouldn't end up on our hips.

Of course, anything that sounds that good has to have a catch. And it does. Olestra acts like a laxative, taking valuable fat-soluble vitamins (A, D, E, and K) and carotenoids with it down the drain. To compensate for the loss, the FDA required that P&G fortify olestra with these nutrients. Not only that, the FDA stipulated that a food containing olestra must include on the label that the product "may cause abdominal cramping and loose stools," and that olestra "inhibits the absorption of some vitamins and other nutrients." The FDA had hoped, by its approval of olestra, that consumers would be able to cut back on fat without sacrificing their favorite foods. In January 1996, the FDA gave the green light for Olean to be included in "savory snacks." The first chips to roll off the assembly line were WOW!Chips by Frito-Lay, followed by P&G's own Pringles. The problem is, consumers have gotten carried away with fat-free foods, eating them with reckless abandon, and never stopping to consider how many calories they're consuming. Calories do count—it's not just the fat that matters.

Olestra wasn't the first artificial fat. There have been others made from proteins, carbohydrates, or fats, which have been made in ways to mimic the feel of fat in your mouth. Simplesse and Avicel, for example, have been used in a variety of foods, including cheese, chips, frozen desserts, and candy. Considering America's desire for pleasure without the fat, these fat substitutes probably won't be the last.

Making the Most of Fat

We eat fatty foods because they taste good and make us feel full. You now know that there are some fats you must have in your diet. If you're going to make the most of the fat you're allowed, here are some suggestions:

1. Be generous with seasonings, so you don't have to rely on fat for flavor.
2. If you're cooking with butter, let it brown in the frying pan first (make sure, though, that you don't let it burn), to increase its flavor intensity and allow you to use less.
3. Select strong-flavored cheeses.
4. Use soup stock in place of fat when sautéing.

5. Select low-fat foods only when the calories are also reduced compared to the full-fat version. Look at the label to find out how much sugar has been added in the low-fat or nonfat variety, as compensation for having the fat removed.

chapter 8

Life Is Uncertain—Eat Dessert First

Seize the moment! Remember all those women on the Titanic who waved off the dessert cart.

—*Erma Bombeck*

America has a love affair with sugar. And this love affair is getting worse. Between 1972 and 1976, we were eating about 123 pounds of sweeteners (sugar, high-fructose corn syrup, and honey) per person per year. In 1999, we had increased that intake to 158 pounds. If you do the math, that's almost ½ pound (or 50 teaspoons) per person per day. Of course, no one is sitting around eating teaspoon after teaspoon of sugar from the sugar bowl (or are you?). Some of the sugar we're eating is obvious—in cakes, candies, and ice cream. However, there's a great deal of sugar we're unaware of—in spaghetti sauce, soups, and condiments, to name a few.

Reading food labels will tell you how much sugar is in a food. The problem is, the amount of sugar listed on the label reflects not only naturally occurring sugars, such as in fruit and milk, but also what's been added. Unfortunately for the

Nutrition Facts	
Serving Size 1 Can	
Amount Per Serving	
Calories 140	
	% Daily Value*
Total Fat 0g	0%
Sodium 50mg	2%
Total Carbohydrate 39g	13%
Sugars 39g	
Protein 0g	

Label for soda.

consumer, food manufacturers aren't required to state how much is "added sugars." Knowing what the food is should help. For example, as you can see from the label to the left, a can of soda is pure sugar, plus carbonated water. On the other hand, it may take some guesswork or looking at the list of ingredients when you're considering other foods. Let's say you're having a glass of chocolate low-fat milk. The label tells you that there are 26 grams of sugars. Compare that to plain low-fat milk with 12 grams of sugars (naturally occurring as lactose). If you subtract the two, you'll see that the sugar added to the chocolate milk amounts to 14 grams.

With that in mind, the next question should be how much added sugar is considered healthy. According to the World Health Organization (WHO), we shouldn't be having more than 10 percent of the total calories we eat coming from added sugars. What does that mean for you personally? In Chapter 16, you'll be finding out how many calories is right for you. When you've found that out, come back here and look at the following table. Keep the number you find in this table in mind as you look at the heading "Sugars" on food labels. As you eat different foods, add up the grams of sugars, being sure not to go over your daily allowance. (With so many foods containing sugar, staying within your limit isn't as easy as it may seem.)

How Much Added Sugar You Can Have

Calorie Allowance	Calories Sugar	Grams Sugar	Teaspoons Sugar
1,200	120	30	8
1,500	150	$37\frac{1}{2}$	10
1,800	180	45	12
2,100	210	$52\frac{1}{2}$	14
2,400	240	60	16

Let's take several foods as examples. Suppose you want to have a can of soda. The label says a 12-ounce can has 140 calories and 39 grams "Sugars." If you're eating 1,500 calories a day, that one can of soda is all the added sugar you can have. But what about the ketchup that you put on your hamburger, which has 4 grams of sugars, or that glass of chocolate milk with the 14 grams added sugar? You've really blown it. In fact, someone on 1,800 and even 2,100 calories has gone over the limit. If you really want a soda, you might want to start drinking diet sodas, especially when research is showing that so many of the extra calories Americans are now consuming come from sodas.

You need to keep in mind that sugar is really nutritionally worthless other than the calories it provides for energy. It gives you no vitamins or minerals. Yet if you have a piece of fruit instead, to satisfy your sweet tooth, you get some energy calories and some nutrition. And you don't have to deduct the grams of sugar in fresh fruit from the total grams of added sugar you're allowed for the day.

Check out Appendix D to get an idea of how many teaspoons of sugar you're getting with some of the foods you eat. I slipped in one main dish to give you a heads-up that many of the prepared entrées you eat are loaded with sugar. To find out how many teaspoons of sugar are in the foods you eat, look at the food label under "Sugars" and divide that number of grams by four.

So you may ask, "If life is uncertain, how can I fit dessert in, when desserts contain a great deal of added sugar?" The answer to that is "sparingly." Yet it is possible. You'll have to think of dessert differently than you have been. Instead of dessert being another course in the meal, it truly is a treat and not something you have to have. When you do have it, consider it in terms of "a taste" rather than slices, cups, or ounces. When you want to have some ice cream, take one tablespoon and nurse it, lick it, savor it, focus on it, make the most of it. If you want some chocolate, consider a teaspoon of fat-free chocolate syrup and treat it the same way as the ice cream. Eat it very *slooowwwwly!* When you have the urge for something sweet, consider eating sweetened breakfast cereals instead of candy or cookies. If you have a cookie, break it in half and save one-half for another time. (Just remember the old law of physics that says breaking a cookie in half lets the calories fall out!) Dried fruit is also a good alternative, because it's sweet and also gives you some nutrition at the same time. Plan ahead. If you know you're going to have cake at a particular occasion, don't have foods with added sugars during the day.

The Art of Tasting

Our desire for sweet things starts at an early age. A baby's tongue has more taste buds than that of an adult, and those taste buds are more sensitive to all the flavors. That's because a baby's tongue hasn't had to put up with the insults of hot food that we, as adults, weren't willing to let cool sufficiently before eating. The taste buds for sweet things are right on the tip of the tongue. Therefore, it's the area that gets the first onslaught of the food's flavor. Anything that's sweet will be readily accepted—for example, mother's milk. This, in some ways, probably starts our training and habit of enjoying sweet things.

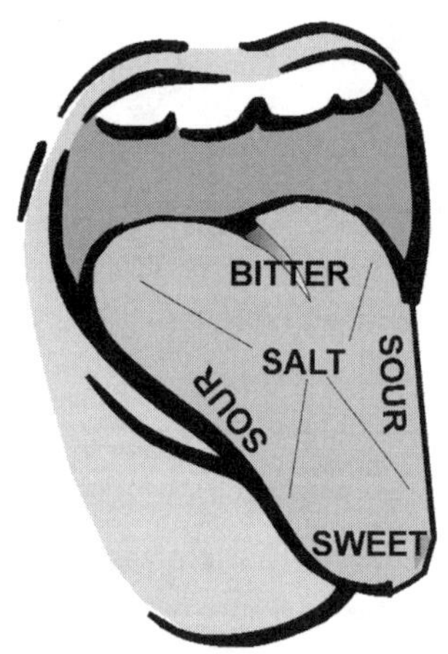

Where we taste things.

Our sensitivity to sweet flavors is the weakest of the taste perceptions, followed by salty flavors, sour flavors, and bitter flavors, which we can detect in very minute amounts. Considering that poisonous substances are normally bitter, it's good that our tongues are that sensitive to bitter flavors. If you look at the diagram of the tongue you'll see that the taste buds for bitter lie at the back. This is nature's way of giving us one last chance to spit something out that might be harmful to our health. It may force us to gag.

Taste buds don't have a long life. About every 10 days, some die off and are replaced. At least, that is, before we turn 45. Then the taste buds are replaced at a slower rate. That might explain why we tend to favor more intense flavors as we get older—we're trying to get the same taste jolt that we had when we were younger. I wonder if that's why we boomers have warmly embraced Mexican and Cajun cooking?

Even if we were to have our tongues cut out, we would still experience some flavors, because there are taste buds on the roof of the mouth, as well as the inside of the cheeks. What would curtail our ability to taste would be the lack of saliva, because the flavors wouldn't be able to dissolve and spread over the taste buds.

Taste is a highly personal thing, because of the variation of sensitivity of the individual tongue. Some people may crave salt, whereas others may be repelled by too much of it. There are those who love the five-alarm hot sauce, whereas others need only sniff the stuff to run for water. Brussels sprouts, with their sulfurous overtones, may smell too noxious for some people to be palatable, whereas other people like the bitter taste.

> The cuisine of countries with warmer climates tends to be spicier than that found in the northern hemisphere. That's because spicy foods tend to make one sweat, which in hot climates actually works to cool the body.

Many of the tastes that we find appealing are based on heredity. In addition, we acquire tastes as we grow older. If that weren't the case, such foods as coffee, hot peppers, and fruits that make you pucker would never be eaten. Offer a lemon to a baby and watch the face it makes. You won't get it to eat too much more. As adults, though, we may find the acidity a nice contrast to iced tea or fish. We're able to enjoy bitter flavors more as we age, which may explain why some vegetables "grow on us." We've learned to eat certain foods because our parents ate them. If we liked them when they were first introduced, we're probably still eating them. On the other hand, if our first encounter wasn't pleasant, it's less likely we'll subject ourselves to the experience again, unless we can see some redeeming value in eating it.

Smell is an integral part of taste. (You know that's true when you have a cold and can't taste a thing.) That's because smell and taste share a common air passage. The smell of food is what hits us first, before we ever taste it. If the smell is enticing, we'll try it. Otherwise, we may just pass. Some people find the smell of fish unpleasant to get past their noses in order for the taste buds to get a chance to make their own decision.

Other qualities of food contribute to its taste and pleasure—its texture, temperature, and appearance. Even the sound it makes as we chew it influences the impression it leaves. A candy called Pop Rocks, that literally explode in your mouth, provides numerous sensations. It's sweet, it's hard at first, and then as it dissolves on your tongue, it makes a crackling sound. You can actually feel the "pop" on your tongue. Although there's nothing nutritionally redeeming about Pop Rocks, it's an example of a food that makes an impression on you. A good crispy potato chip has a similar effect.

Chewing is also an important part of taste. The slower you eat something, the more time you give the food to roll around over all the various taste buds. That way you can experience the full extent of the flavors—from sweet to salty to sour to bitter. If you do chew slowly, you'll appreciate why texture plays such a large part of the sensory experience of a food. If all the food we ate were in the consistency of pudding, we'd grow bored with eating, because everything could be swallowed instantaneously, with no time for the flavors to register on the taste buds. What titillates the taste buds is not only the flavor, but also the crunchiness and chewiness of the food.

> When I watch dogs eat, I wonder how they can find any pleasure from their food. Most dogs wolf down their meal, leaving little time for the taste buds to experience the flavor. (Whenever you're tempted to eat that way, you might as well set a bowl of food on the floor and get down on all fours to eat!)

Let's do a chocolate taste test to see how to experience flavor. What we do here with chocolate may be done with any food, not just sweets. To make this experiment work, you need to be fully focused on the process. Start by choosing a good-quality chocolate. Look for one with a high percentage of chocolate liquor. Belgian chocolate, in my opinion, is the best.

- Look at the chocolate. Is the surface velvety, shiny, or does it have a matte finish? (Remember, appearance of food either tantalizes and tempts or detracts and repels.)
- Break the chocolate. What sound does it produce? Did it snap or just break quietly?
- Smell the aroma. Do you get a strong chocolatey smell or somewhat more waxy?

- Put the piece of chocolate on your tongue and experience the mouth feel. Don't chew it. Let it start to melt on your tongue. Does it have a smooth, rich consistency or somewhat gritty?
- Experience the flavor. Allow the chocolate to roll around in your mouth, experiencing not only the front and top of the tongue, but the sides, under the tongue, the roof of your mouth, and your cheeks. Don't swallow just yet. Think about the flavors you're sensing. Are they nutty and roasted, mingling with sweetness?

Think about this kind of tasting experience when you sit down to eat, no matter what the food. Try to concentrate on what you're eating and why you're receiving pleasure, if any, from it. My hope is that you'll slow down your eating process and receive more taste fulfillment from less. By not overeating, you'll help yourself to lose weight.

It's hard to separate the emotional attachment people have to chocolate from the chemical action it has on the body. Chocolate is both a stimulant and a relaxant. It contains theobromine, a mild caffeinelike substance. Being a carbohydrate, it also stimulates the production of serotonin in the brain, which has a calming effect. Maybe chocolate cravings aren't just in our heads. The chocolate industry is trying to convince us that its antioxidant activity gives chocolate some health benefits. However, those antioxidants come at a very high-fat, high-sugar, and high-calorie price.

The reputation of chocolate as a food of love and romance may have nothing to do with what nutrients it contains. Give credit to the candy companies that have made it a tradition for such occasions as Valentine's Day and Mother's Day. Better yet, give credit to the Aztecs, the Indians of Central and South America, who considered it so special that only the rulers were allowed to indulge in this gift of the god, Quetzalcoatl. However, I don't think any of us chocolate lovers would have enjoyed the way chocolate was originally served. It was made into a thick drink, without sugar, and often spiked with hot peppers.

Sugar Aliases

A sugar by another name is still sugar—empty calories. When you look at the list of ingredients in food, you may not realize where the sugar is lurking. Keep an eye out for the following:

- Beet sugar
- Brown sugar
- Cane sugar
- Confectioner's sugar
- Crystallized cane juice
- Dextrin
- Dextrose
- Evaporated cane juice
- Fructose
- High-fructose corn syrup
- Honey
- Invert sugar
- Levulose
- Maltodextrin
- Maple syrup
- Molasses
- Raw sugar
- Sucrose
- Table sugar
- Turbinado sugar
- White sugar

Sorbitol, mannitol, and xylitol are sugar alcohols that have slightly fewer calories than regular sugar. At least they don't cause the spikes in insulin that can occur with regular sugar. Keep in mind that ingredients on a food label are listed in descending order of weight—the ingredient with the most weight being listed first. Clever food manufacturers have figured out how to fool us, whether intentionally or not. By including in a food several different forms of sugar, no single type may have enough weight to put it at the top of the list. From just a quick glance at the ingredients, you're led to believe that there isn't that much sugar in the product. But if you'll take a few extra moments to notice how many times you see a sugar mentioned in the list of ingredients, you'll see how they can add up to the amount of sugar shown on the label's Nutrition Facts.

The biggest problem with too much sugar in a person's diet is that it crowds out good nutrition. Who has enough room for vegetables, fruits, and whole grains when they've filled up on sweets? Think about what your mother used to tell you when you were younger. "Don't eat that candy before dinner. It'll spoil your appetite." Our mothers were very smart. We're the fools if we're not listening.

Pretty Sweet Deal

Thanks to several twists of fate, we now have sugar substitutes that were not originally destined for the sugar bowl. *Saccharin*, which was discovered in 1879 at Johns Hopkins University, was probably the first of the non-nutritive sweeteners. The product was initially intended as an antiseptic and food preservative. With the sugar shortage during World War II, saccharin stepped in to fill the void. Everyone probably knows saccharin as the "pink packet" of sweetener from Sweet'N Low.

Because we obviously use sugar substitutes in place of sugar, we tend to measure the sweetness of a substitute against pure sugar. Saccharin, for example, is 300 to 500 times as sweet as sugar. Some people find saccharin's astringent, bitter, and metallic aftertaste unappealing. However, for many years it gave people with diabetes a sweetener that didn't affect their insulin levels, and gave dieters a way to enjoy a sweet taste without any calories. Unfortunately, in 1972, it was taken off the FDA's generally recognized as safe (GRAS) list due to studies showing it caused bladder cancer in rats. There was concern that there could be a possible correlation to humans. Even though the FDA revoked its ban against saccharin in 1977, it required the product to carry a warning about possible bladder cancer. Finally, in 2000, the FDA gave saccharin a clean bill of health, no longer requiring the warning message. Considering its checkered past, it's up to you to decide whether you feel comfortable eating products with saccharin. The reason many people lean toward saccharin over other sugar substitutes is price.

Saccharin's archrival is *aspartame,* the "blue packet" sold under the name NutraSweet or Equal. It tastes approximately 180 to 200 times sweeter than sugar. Here again, we have a product that was being developed for a purpose other than as a sweetener. G.D. Searle & Co. was looking for a product for ulcer therapy, combining two amino acids, phenylalanine and aspartic acid. The chemist tasted the product and found it amazingly sweet. In 1981, the FDA approved aspartame as safe, except for people with phenylketonuria, a condition where the body can't break down phenylalanine. After the problems the FDA encountered with saccharin, the FDA did rigorous testing before allowing the product to be sold. The FDA states that 50 milligrams aspartame per kilogram of body weight is an acceptable daily intake (ADI). For example, a 150-pound adult could drink 20 (12-ounce) containers of soda or eat 42 (4-ounce) servings of sugar-free gelatin or consume 97 packets of sweetener—and still be fine. Most people don't even come close to the ADI. Some people say they get an adverse reaction from aspartame, such as a headache or upset stomach. If you have problems with the product, there are numerous others on the market that might work for you.

Acesulfame (*ace-sul-fame*) *potassium,* also known as acesulfame-K, is 200 times sweeter than sugar. It's marketed under the brand names of Sunett and Sweet One. The advantage it has over aspartame is that it can be used in baking and cooking without breaking down. However, the end product isn't quite as good as that made with pure sugar.

Another sugar substitute is a product called *sucralose* marketed as Splenda. It's approximately 600 times sweeter than sugar and, like acesulfame-K, it's heat stable. Even though it's made from sugar, the body doesn't recognize it as a carbohydrate, so it goes through the digestive tract unchanged and is eliminated. The ADI established by the FDA is 5 milligrams per kilogram of body weight per day.

It's nice to have noncaloric sweeteners that allow you to indulge your sweet tooth without the calories. However, these are substances put together in a chemistry lab, and you're asking your body to deal with them as if they're natural. My recommendation is, first of all, limit the amount of these artificial substances you eat. Second, strive toward eating a healthier, more natural diet, which includes foods with less processing. Third, when you want something sweet, learn to enjoy nature's bounty of fruits. Finally, train your taste buds to enjoy less intensity of sugar, just as your palate can be educated to like less fatty foods.

part 2

What's a Person to Believe?

Have you been lured into trying new diets because the advertisements and stories that are told sound too good to pass up? Actually, once you know the truth behind these diets, you'll appreciate how many of those stories sound too good to be true. Losing weight takes time. Yet we're so easily attracted to the promises of instant success and quick weight loss. And understandably so, because most people who find themselves in an uncomfortable position try to get out of it as rapidly as possible. Just as it took you some time to gain the weight, losing it may take just as long. In this section, I share with you the many diet products we boomers have encountered as we've grown up. One of the more popular diets today is the high-protein diet (most notable being the Atkins Diet). I believe that anyone who chooses to do this or any diet should have an understanding of how the body deals with the food they eat. If you know what happens to that food, you are in a better position to more wisely select that food. I hope that after you read this section you'll reconsider some of the choices you're making.

chapter 9

Growing Up with Diet Products

There are some remedies worse than the disease.
—Publilius Syrus

Just when did it become fashionable to be thin? One might say it was in the early 1920s, when the flapper look was in. Trying to achieve a somewhat boyish figure, women corseted themselves to a point where their breasts hardly showed. With their dresses hanging straight and flat, they could wear a very long necklace of beads and not have to worry that, as they moved, the necklace would slip over one breast or the other. Even further back in time, women wore corsets in an attempt to make their waists appear very small and accentuate their busts. Personally, I'm glad we gave up the corsets. Those women were constantly passing out, because they could not take a deep enough breath to get enough oxygen. During the 1970s, the women's liberation movement started a "burn the bra" campaign to symbolize that liberation. ("Free at last!")

It didn't last long, but that's typical of how fashion swings back and forth like the pendulum of a grandfather clock. We've passed from the flapper look to Marilyn Monroe, back to Twiggy, and now to folks like Niki Taylor, Heidi Klum, Naomi Campbell, Elle MacPherson, and Antonio Sabato Jr. (who models for Calvin Klein). Although men have probably always wanted to look fit, looking thin wasn't part of their image. (That's especially true of the wealthy in the nineteenth century, who showed how much they had by how much they could eat.) Today men have become more concerned about weight, not just muscle mass. So they, too, have taken to dieting.

> *When the women's liberation movement started, I was the first to burn my bra. It took three days to put out the fire.*
>
> —*Dolly Parton*

Our lives seem centered around food, so it's not surprising to see the problem our country has with obesity. Social events aren't complete without food. The meaning of the holidays becomes lost under the weight of the foods that are served. Birthdays, promotions, pay raises, and anything that can be celebrated is done with food. People go out for dinner or raise a toast to commemorate the event. Don't get me wrong. I'm all for celebrating, but not at the sake of our health.

The way people try to have their cake and eat it too is to enjoy themselves eating, suffer the consequence of gaining weight, then pay the price by dieting it off. And the weight-loss industry is more than happy to help. What often astounds me is that people are willing to pay hundreds and hundreds of dollars on pills, potions, and gadgets, but consider it frivolous and too expensive to see a registered dietitian who's trained to help people lose weight. They're probably afraid that a dietitian will tell them something they don't want to hear or don't want to do; whereas pills, potions, and gadgets seem like a quick fix, and saves being embarrassed. Read on and you decide.

In Search of the Magic Bullet

Pop a pill and you will see instant results. No need to change your eating habits. No need to exercise.

How can so many people be fooled so much of the time? I know that people who are overweight will jump on any train that's going to Never-Be-Fat-Again Land. The wish that it all could be gone overnight makes many people suckers for the diet industry's booming business. There have been diet patches worn on the skin, even though the FDA did not approve these. The "fat blockers" purport to physically absorb fat and mechanically interfere with the fat a person eats. The "starch blockers" promise similar results except that they work on carbohydrates instead of fat. It sounds like a great idea if only it worked. It doesn't. Instead, you can end up with a terrible case of diarrhea and stomach pains, possibly resulting in a drop of electrolytes, which can be harmful to your health. It doesn't sound to me like the smartest way to lose weight. Besides, why eat something and not have it absorbed. Remember, the reason for eating is to nourish the body.

When I was young the first appetite suppressant I remember was a product called Ayds, little chocolate squares. Since then the market has been inundated with over-the-counter appetite suppressants. You've probably heard of some of them: Acutrim, Dexatrim, herbal PhenFen, and Xenadrine. Garcinia has gotten attention lately. It contains hydroxycitric acid that purportedly burns fat. There need to be more studies done to prove whether it is safe and effective.

> Ephedrine is derived from an herb called ephedra, also known as *ma huang*.

The pills, though, that have been grabbing attention in the news lately are ephedrine based.

Ephedrine is a component of adrenaline and has similar effects in some people—rapid heartbeat, high blood pressure, heart attack, stroke, and seizures. Some deaths have even resulted from the products. One notable fatality occurred on February 19, 2003, when Baltimore Orioles pitching prospect Steve Bechler died of heatstroke in Fort Lauderdale, Florida. He'd been taking a weight-loss drug that contained ephedrine. The fact that ephedrine has been banned by the NCAA, NFL, and the International Olympic Committee should send a red flag up for those who want to try it. Having high blood pressure or heart disease should be another warning sign. Among the most popular of these ephedrine-based pills are Metabolife and Herbalife. Unless users change their lifestyle habits, none of these pills works. Taking a pill is really a crutch—where users come to depend upon its powers. In reality, the power to change lies within ourselves.

Another questionable compound is phenylpropanolamine, which has been used in diet drugs to control appetite. A study done at Yale University in May 2000 led the FDA to request that drug companies no longer make products with phenylpropanolamine. A few of the people in the study suffered hemorrhagic strokes.

The Prescription Approach

When you're taking prescription drugs for weight loss, at least you're under the guidance of a physician who can keep track of how your body reacts to the medication. None of these diet pills is without potential risks. Meridia is supposed to make you feel full because it modulates two brain chemicals—serotonin and norepinephrine. Serotonin controls appetite, whereas norepinephrine is involved in metabolism. Side effects range from a minor dry mouth to concern that the drug can affect heart rate and blood pressure. A major drawback to Meridia is that, when discontinued, there can be significant weight regain.

Products like Redux and Pondimin, which contain fenfluramine, were developed to increase the availability of serotonin in the brain. Fenfluramine supposedly reduces calorie intake because of its effect on serotonin's control of the appetite center in the brain. You may be familiar with the combination drug referred to as Fen/Phen (a combination of fenfluramine and phentermine). The media brought the public's attention to the product in the mid-1990s. At that time it was being sold as "the answer to our problems." In a late 1990s study of women taking Fen/Phen, the Mayo Clinic found that participants had developed valvular heart disease. These were women who had no previous history of cardiac problems. At the request of the FDA, Redux, Pondimin, and Fen/Phen were taken off the market. As it turns out, it was the combination of the two substances that caused the problem. It's thought that fenfluramine was the culprit. Because of its 30-year history of success as a diet drug in Europe, phentermine has remained on the market for short-term use.

Then there are liquid diets that are supervised by physicians. They include Medifast, the Cambridge Diet, and Optifast. In 1988 the public became aware of Optifast (from Sandoz Nutrition) when Oprah Winfrey, the television talk-show host, went on the diet. The audience was glued to their sets every day to watch the 70 pounds melt away. Unfortunately, it didn't last, because the most important component of losing weight and maintaining that loss is establishing a healthy relationship to food and, without question, to exercise.

People are now holding out hope for a hormone called *leptin*—a protein produced naturally in the body in adipose (fat) tissue. It travels to the brain where it inhibits food intake by its interaction with neurotransmitters. As a therapeutic agent, the idea would be to inject leptin into obese people and let it help suppress appetite. However, researchers are finding that it's not that obese people are deficient in leptin, but that they are insensitive to it. So more research needs to be done to find ways to overcome the resistance. One thing that has been found is that after people have lost weight, their level of leptin goes down, possibly triggering increased hunger and a slower metabolism. If that's the case, it means that after you lose weight, you need to be even more diligent with controlling the amount you eat. Smaller meals more often will help you control your hunger. In addition, increasing your exercise will help rev up your metabolism.

Sip a Shake

Most of you are probably familiar with Slim-Fast and its liquid meal-replacement program. There are other similar products, such as Nestle Sweet Success and Ensure. To lose weight, they recommend you drink two meal-replacement beverages and eat a sensible dinner. These beverages weren't the first liquid diet on the market. Do you remember Metracal? It was introduced in the 1950s, predating Slim-Fast by many years. The manufacturers of the product suggested replacing only your lunch with Metracal, so people who used the product were called the "Metracal for Lunch Bunch." I even remember my mother trying Metracal. She didn't stick to it for very long because, as is true for most people, chewing is an important part of the enjoyment of a meal. There was also a diet drink by Pet Milk called Sego. (An interesting fact is that when Alfred Hitchcock saw Tippi Hedren doing a commercial for Sego, he decided to cast her in his thriller *The Birds.*) One thing you can say for liquid meal replacements is that they're easy—there's no assembly required. They can also be grabbed and consumed on the run. I have to admit as I'm writing this, I'm cringing. I find it really sad that we can't find the time to sit down to eat a decent meal. I often question our priorities.

Your first and foremost reason for eating should be to nourish your body. If you don't feed it, it won't run. It's that simple. Beyond that, many of us eat for the pleasure of the experience. So whenever you start to put something in your mouth, ask yourself if it's something that will be good for your body. Then ask yourself whether you're truly enjoying it.

> For me, anything I eat had better be enjoyable. Otherwise, it isn't worth the calories.

Count, Count, Count

Counting calories and grams of fat have been very popular approaches to losing weight. You could buy little pocket books that gave you the calories and fat grams of food, so that you'd always have the information with you when you had to make a decision on what to eat. Then people became creative and designed fat wheels. These were little cardboard gadgets with two circles attached at their centers, allowing you to spin one against the other. The Fat Finder was one such wheel. The top circle had grams of fat shown in tick marks around the circumference, ranging in value from 1.5 grams to 60 grams fat. The bottom circle was larger and showed total calories, ranging from 10 to 600. From information you could find on a food label, you'd line up the tick mark of the grams of fat in the food with the mark showing the total number of calories. The percentage of fat in the food would show in the window. At the time, anything more than 30 percent was considered a no-no because the government had said we should be eating less than 30 percent of our total calories from fat. This was misinterpreted as meaning one food by itself should not have more than

30 percent of calories from fat. That's not what was meant, because certain foods like oil, for example, are 100 percent fat. This misinterpretation would mean that healthy oils such as olive oil would have to be eliminated. However, it did make people more aware of what they were eating. And it was fun to "spin the wheel."

Number counting is now the basis of the Weight Watcher's Winning Points Plan. Instead of a wheel, you have something called a Points Finder. A cardboard sleeve with a slider lets you line up numbers for calories, fiber, and total fat to get the points for a food. Before you start the diet, you're given the total number of points you're allowed for your calorie level. It's interesting that during the 1990s, no one wanted to count calories. They had done enough of that in the 1970s and 1980s, and were happy to give it up. Yet we now know that calories do count, and need to be considered when determining how much you can eat for the day.

Gadgets and Gizmos

We are one lazy society. Given the choice, we'd rather let a machine do the work, any work, than have to exert ourselves. Consider all the modern conveniences we have, from electric lawn mowers (they even have one now that works by remote control) to portable phones that people hook onto their belts. Manufacturers took that mind-set to the weight-loss industry and found a ready market. Do you remember when you were a kid, seeing one of those vibrator machines? The gadget was about two to three feet wide, and the motor was about waist high off the ground on a pedestal. Attached at each side of the motor was the end of a five-inch wide leather belt. Users would step inside the belt, slipping it around their butt or waist. Then they'd flip a switch and the belt started to vibrate. The idea was that you could jiggle the fat off. Unfortunately, you don't lose fat that way. Losing fat requires that you lose weight and build muscle. Of course, when you got finished with the vibrator, you had pretty tender fat. It just reinforced the fallacy that you can spot reduce. While the machine may not have done much for the user, it was quite amusing for an outside observer to watch all that flab jiggle. That gadget appeared in any number of cartoons and spoofs in the movies and on TV.

Another product that was based on the idea of spot reduction was the cream you could put on your thighs to eliminate cellulite. That's the dimply or lumpy appearance the skin has (which women so affectionately called "cottage cheese") because of underlying fat. There was also the neoprene waist belt that would shrink the fat cells around your waist, and the neoprene shorts to thin out your thighs. Let me say right now that you cannot take fat off in specific areas. You can only lose weight and let your body decide what fat stores it wants to get rid of. By the way, the place your body takes the fat off first probably won't be where you'd want to lose it first!

Another device that used the same philosophy was a roller-type machine. It looked like a free-standing radiator whose top center section revolved. Someone using the machine would lean over the revolving section, allowing the abdomen to make contact with the machine. As the section moved, the abdomen would be massaged—in the hope that the fat would disappear. Are you familiar with Kobe beef? The cows are massaged daily, which makes the meat very tender. That's pretty much what someone using the above machine was doing—they were becoming tender meat, not *lean* meat.

Then there was the sauna suit. It was a space-age-looking outfit made of some sort of silver reflective fabric. When you put it on, you looked like you were wrapped in aluminum foil. The concept behind it was to sweat the fat off. After using the suit, people got on their scales to happily find they had indeed lost weight. What they'd really lost was water, which, of course, is not a permanent weight-loss solution. There were also steam cabinets, popular when we were kids, which used the same sweat-it-off philosophy, as do the steam rooms today. You'll come out relaxed, but no less fat.

You Gotta Get a Gimmick

In the musical *Gypsy,* one of the fun numbers is called "You Gotta Get a Gimmick … If You're Gonna Get Ahead." I think a good number of weight-loss companies took that song to heart. They make the process of losing weight appear so effortless that you'd be a fool not to try it. It's amusing to listen to the claims and promises they make. "Lose fat while you sleep!" "Eat all you want and still lose weight!" "The fat will just melt away!" They're all nonsense, but that little exclamation point after each claim actually makes you want to believe it and gets you excited to try. Some companies use celebrities to push their products. Weight Watchers, for example, uses Sarah Ferguson, the Duchess of York.

In the 1990s, "appetite-suppressing eyeglasses" were popular. They were like common eyeglasses with colored lenses that claimed to project an image to the retina that dampened the desire to eat. Some of them were made with a color that made your food look so obnoxious you wouldn't want to eat it. Because there isn't any evidence to back up the effectiveness of these glasses, I suppose that product died a quiet death. I haven't heard any more about them. It's interesting how you hear about a new product everywhere you turn—until the truth gets out that it really doesn't work. Then it just slowly and quietly disappears. Never fear, though, there is sure to be another product in its wake. Another interesting product is called "magic weight-loss earrings." The idea behind these is to stimulate acupuncture points in the ear that control hunger. It hasn't been proven to be helpful, but it does sound like an intriguing concept.

That brings me to a very important point. Anything that's truly effective should be able to stand up to rigorous studies conducted by qualified researchers. Double-blind studies are the best, because then neither the researcher nor the subjects know who's getting the real thing and who's getting a placebo. (A placebo, sometimes called a "sugar pill," is a dummy treatment given in place of a real treatment, to test that the real treatment works significantly better than nothing at all.)

Then there are the diets that claim you can lose weight in five days or seven days. You'll be lucky if you can lose one to two pounds in five or seven days. There's no way you're going to lose any more than that safely.

Here are some words used in product claims that sound too good to be true—most often, they're not:

- Amazing
- Ancient
- Breakthrough
- Easy
- Effortless
- Exclusive
- Exotic
- Fast working

- Guaranteed
- Immediate
- Magical
- Miraculous
- Mysterious
- Natural
- New discovery
- Painless
- Panacea
- Revolutionary
- Secret formula

Can We Talk?

Some of the diet approaches I've discussed so far are either outlandish, faddish, or have no basis in research to prove them either effective or safe. However, there are some approaches that are. One of those is group support, which has been around for a long time. In fact, Weight Watchers began in September 1961, when Jean Nidetch, who was overweight, invited a group of friends over to her house, confessing to them that she had an eating obsession. She couldn't keep from eating cookies—they were her downfall. Having the comfort of her friends helped her lose 70 pounds, and her program became one of the most successful weight-control organizations in the world. By May 1963, Weight Watchers was doing so well that it incorporated. Through the years, behavior modification and exercise have been added to the program. They also started making foods to sell in grocery stores.

What Jean realized is that people often need the group support and empathy of others to address why they're eating the way they are or gaining weight. Most people don't choose to be fat. Life often takes them that way because of the stresses they encounter or the households in which they grew up. Other organizations have tried to address this group-support need—TOPS (Take Off Pounds Sensibly), KOPS (Keep Off Pounds Sensibly), and Overeaters Anonymous. For people wanting some one-on-one attention, there's Jenny Craig and Diet Centers. However, one of the requirements of these organizations is to buy their food. That may be good news for people who don't like to cook or don't have time to. However, it can be very expensive.

chapter 10

The Allure of Fad Diets

Thank you for calling the Weight Loss Hotline.
If you'd like to lose a half-pound right now, press "1" eighteen thousand times.
—*Randy Glasbergen*

How many diets have you tried? The average American has probably tried at least one or two, if not more. Note that I didn't say how many times has the average American tried to lose weight. That number would be much greater. The term *yo-yo dieting* didn't come about for nothing. Diets seem to come and go out of style just like clothes. Do you remember the bell-bottom pants we wore? When those went out of fashion, I never believed they would return. They're back, and so have many diets of yesteryear resurfaced. How exciting. We have a new diet to try.

You have to admit that there is an allure to a "new" diet, where not only its creator but the media tout how great it is. Advertisers are sure to show you the before and after pictures to prove how successful people can be on a particular plan. Have you ever noticed, though, in the fine print at the bottom of the television screen or ad, it says that these results are not typical? I suppose they figure that because they're appealing to us baby boomers, our eyesight is such that we wouldn't be able to read the fine print without our glasses anyway. They play on our sense of optimism, a hope that this time this diet will be the one. The fact is, people can lose weight on almost any diet. The question is, for how long? I'll be reviewing some of the popular diets to point out their shortcomings and give you some thoughts on how to know what is the best way to lose weight. I normally recommend to my clients something that is healthy, something that is easy to follow, and something that you can do for the rest of your life. It's not glamorous or faddish, but it's simple and works.

The One-Food or Specific-Food Approach

For a while, the ***Cabbage Soup Diet*** was popular. The concept behind it is you can eat as much cabbage soup as you want, but nothing else. People did lose weight on it. Why? After days and days of the same flavor, they couldn't stand the thought of eating any more. Sheer boredom and taste fatigue set in.

The author, Margaret Danbrot, wanted readers to believe that there was some magical property in cabbage that would help burn off the fat. There isn't. The dieters may have been getting their vegetables, but they weren't getting balanced nutrition—the diet lacked protein and other complex carbohydrates beside vegetables. What many people did get from this diet, though, was a lot of flatulence from all that cabbage. Don't get me wrong. I'm all for eating soup, but as part of a meal. In fact, if you want to eat less during the meal, have a broth-based soup as a starter. It helps send signals to the brain that food is on its way and starts to ease the hunger pangs. The problem with this diet, besides that fact that is nutritionally unbalanced, is that it doesn't teach you how to eat healthy.

> The criterion I use to determine a good diet is whether it teaches me how to eat for a lifetime. I don't want to have to learn to eat one way during the diet, only to have to change my approach when I reach my goal weight. As we all know, habits are hard to break. (And we're old enough to have created a number of them.) New habits are even harder to make. So why learn one set of habits for the diet and then have to learn another set for maintaining the weight you lost?

Another diet that concentrates on specific foods is the ***New Beverly Hills Diet*** by Judy Mazel and Michael Wyatt. This diet had been around for a long time under the name the Beverly Hills Diet, but lost favor when many people tried it, got severe cases of diarrhea and dehydration, and had to see their doctor. However, it was brought back when fad diets seemed to have picked up in popularity. With a name like New Beverly Hills Diet, it sounds like something all the celebrities are trying. I hope that doesn't tempt you.

The idea behind this diet is if you don't carefully combine certain foods, and instead eat freely from all groups of foods, you'll gain weight. The authors say that it is only with specific food combinations that the enzymes in your body can function properly. If you do it wrong, the food calories you eat will be stored as fat. That means that you can't mix protein, carbohydrates, and fat in the same meal. The authors believe that by mixing nutrients, such as protein with carbohydrates, the specific enzymes can't get to the targeted nutrients and break them down. That isn't how the body works. If it were, there's next to nothing we could eat, considering most foods are a combination of nutrients. For example, a steak is high in protein and fat. About the only thing we could eat that is a pure nutrient is table sugar!

The authors want you to eat copious amounts of fruit, believing it to have cleansing properties. After a bout of diarrhea, you may feel like you have been cleansed, when what has really happened is that you've lost valuable electrolytes and fluids. Not a smart thing to do. What the authors miss is the fact that there is a benefit in combining foods. For example, if you eat a piece of fruit or a tomato that is high in vitamin C along with vegetables like spinach that contain iron, you'll increase the amount of iron that is absorbed from these foods. Combining foods also slows down the absorption of carbohydrates, resulting in a more consistent level of blood sugar.

Did you ever try the diet ***Eat Right 4 Your Type?*** Talk about a diet taking the world by storm, but one based on a theory that has not been documented in scientific circles. You may think what difference does it make if other scientists have or have not confirmed the premise behind the diet, as long as it works. Therein lies the problem with many diets.

They often make suggestions that could actually be harmful to your health. It's only through scientific corroboration, where others in the field have substantiated the premise, that you can feel more confident in following a diet approach. You may lose weight but become nutritionally deficient. Because the body can compensate for a long time on poor nutrition, it could be years before you actually see the results of what you did. This applies to the Cabbage Soup Diet and the New Beverly Hills Diet, as it does with any diet that suggests you give up certain foods.

Peter D'Adamo, N.D., the author of *Eat Right,* proposes that people use their blood type as the basis for determining what foods they should and should not eat. He says eating foods appropriate for your blood type decreases your risk for the major diseases. Therefore, some people should be vegetarians, shunning meat and dairy products, whereas others should concentrate on meat as the staple of their diet. However, it's not your blood type but your genetic makeup that will influence your potential for certain diseases. (Lifestyle habits also play a part.) For example, if your parents or grandparents died of heart disease, you have a higher risk of getting the disease because of your genes, not your blood type. I would certainly worry, for example, about the recommendation made to people with Type O blood who have heart disease. They're told to eat plenty of animal protein, which, by the way, is loaded with saturated fat. We know that saturated fat is one of the culprits involved in heart disease. This approach is setting someone up for possible disaster.

> If you've gone on any of these diets, you're not doomed to poor health. I just wouldn't continue on them indefinitely. Instead, start making some healthy choices now from what you learn in this book.

The problem with the Eat Right 4 Your Type diet is that it eliminates too many healthy foods. I hope one message you'll take away from this book is the importance of variety. Each food has it owns nutritional profile, and only by eating a variety of foods can you be certain of getting the maximum amount of nutrition available. As adult baby boomers, we have even more variety available to us than we had as children. Take advantage of it.

An Emphasis on Protein

Probably one of the most popular diets today is the ***Dr. Atkins New Diet Revolution.*** As I mentioned earlier about diets coming back in another package, this is one of those diets. It's based on the ketogenic diet of the late 1960s, a time when we were young and most of us didn't have to worry about losing weight. The diet was based on the concept that fat, rather than carbohydrates, would be used for energy. Men are especially attracted to this diet because Dr. Atkins suggests people can eat as much protein and fat as they want, staying away from carbohydrates (other than in the form of a few vegetables). It's understandable why a diet like this is so attractive to some people. Who wouldn't accept an invitation to a free-for-all, getting to eat as much steak, eggs, bacon, cheese, and butter as they wanted?

Without including carbohydrates in the diet for energy, the body must go after its own fat stores. Sounds like heaven. Eat as much meat as you want and burn fat at the same time. There's a catch, though. For the body to process all the ketones formed from using fat as the energy source, the kidneys have to work overtime. As baby boomers, we aren't getting any younger. In addition, as we get older, the kidneys naturally don't function as effectively. Why age them faster than is necessary? It's also surprising how many people are willing to put up with the bad breath that happens with a ketogenic diet, along with possible headaches, constipation, and fatigue.

Because Atkins doesn't make any recommendations regarding the type of fat to eat, one could eat far more saturated fat than is considered healthy. By allowing you as much meat and fatty products as you want, you're sure to eat too much saturated fat. In fact, this diet could be called the high-fat diet/high-protein diet, considering that a person on this diet would be eating upward of 50 percent of the calories from fat. I have to concede one point to this diet and that is, people who go on the diet tend to be less hungry. It does satisfy the appetite. But at what price? I'll be talking more about high-protein diets in the next chapter, so you can decide.

It would be unfair to discuss high-protein diets and not include ***The Zone.*** It, too, suggests eating more protein than that proposed in the

Food Guide Pyramid. The Food Guide Pyramid recommends that Americans eat 50 to 55 percent of their daily calories from carbohydrates, 15 percent from protein, and 30 percent from fat. Barry Sears, Ph.D., believes that every meal should consist of a 40–30–30 ratio; that is, 40 percent of total calories coming from carbohydrates, 30 percent from protein, and 30 percent fat. If people can eat according to this ratio, he believes they'll be able to stay "in the zone." That's where, supposedly, the maximum amount of metabolic calorie burn can occur. Sears and other food manufacturers have been kind enough to offer us products that would maintain that ratio, realizing few Americans would have the patience to calculate everything they ate. Yet it gets us to be dependent upon manufactured foods rather than whole foods.

To give you an idea of how this diet works, let's say that you want to have some crackers for an afternoon snack. Whether you want it or not, you have to have some source of protein (cheese, meat, and so on) to maintain the correct 40–30–30 nutrient ratio. Sometimes you end up eating many more calories than you need just so you can stay "in the zone." In his favor, this plan of Sears helps promote a more balanced approach to eating (albeit a slightly higher level of protein than necessary) over the plan of Dr. Atkins. There is no magic bullet here, though. The reason you're losing weight on this and other high-protein plans is strictly due to the low calorie intake.

> The lower the calorie intake, the greater the weight loss. It's just that simple. No matter what combination of nutrients in the diet, fewer calories leads to weight loss.

Because the high-protein, low-carbohydrate diet became so popular, many others wanted to jump on the bandwagon. There are too many to discuss in depth, but you might have heard of the ***Carbohydrate Addict's Diet*** and ***Protein Power,*** which are also very popular. The problem with most of these high-protein diets is the uncontrolled amount of fat and lack of attention to the type of fat consumed. What they do have going in their favor is they help people break the habit of eating refined carbohydrates, even though they also sacrifice complex carbohydrates in the bargain.

An Emphasis on Carbohydrates

The only nutrient we have left to tweak is fat, replacing it with carbohydrates. Dr. John McDougall, author of ***McDougall Program for Maximum Weight Loss,*** and Dean Ornish, M.D., in his book ***Eat More, Weigh Less,*** recommend that people basically eat a high-fiber vegetarian plan. Dr. Ornish's approach allows the dieter no more than 10 percent of daily calories coming from fat. (Remember, the Food Guide Pyramid recommends 30 percent, making this is a very, very low-fat plan.) He had studied patients with heart disease who, when following the Eat More diet (along with exercise and stress reduction), were able to reverse their condition.

You would have to be very dedicated to follow this diet indefinitely. With it being so low in fat, people are often hungry a short time after a meal. With there being no restriction on the quantity of food you're allowed to eat, you can always eat some more vegetables if you get hungry. One of the positive facets to this diet is a feeling that, with the exception of fat and meat, you can eat unlimited quantities of food. No measuring. No counting calories.

Drinking Your Meals

No discussion of diets would be complete without mentioning ***liquid diets*** such as Slim-Fast. For those people who don't have a lot of time to cook, or the inclination to do so, a liquid meal replacement may seem like the answer. The shakes have added vitamins, minerals, and, in some cases, fiber. However, as you will see later in the book, whole foods pack a nutrition punch that cannot be replaced by supplements. And that's what Slim-Fast is—a beverage spiked with supplements.

When Slim-Fast first came out, it was much like the food-specific diets we discussed earlier. All you got for two of your meals was a liquid shake. How boring does that get? Besides, how much mouth satisfaction is there when all you get to do is drink your meals? Part of the pleasure of eating is the chewing process. If all we had to do were sip our food, we wouldn't need teeth. Slim-Fast came to realize that people weren't really enjoying just drinking their meals. Their response was nutrition bars.

However, because most bars have a candy coating, one has to question whether they're really a meal replacement or a glorified candy bar. To be fair, Slim-Fast does recommend you eat a sensible dinner. Hmmm! If you can eat sensibly for dinner, why can't you do the same thing for breakfast and lunch? Okay, for some the convenience of a meal-in-a-can overtakes other considerations.

I just don't think you should view this as a lifetime approach to eating. Some people have lost weight on Slim-Fast, though I've met many who couldn't stick with it because it didn't satisfy their hunger. Have you noticed the Slim-Fast ads on television, showing slim people having loads of energy and an accompanying statement telling you how much the individual has lost? They say in fine print "These results aren't typical." Then my question is, "What can you expect?" The problem with Slim-Fast is that no lifetime lessons are learned. To be on a Slim-Fast diet is saying it's okay to eat a candy bar for breakfast and one for lunch as long as you eat a healthy dinner. However, the likelihood of getting your required three to five servings of vegetables a day in your one sensible meal is slim.

> Do you know what will be the biggest problem after you've lost weight? You'll have nothing to talk about at cocktail parties or coffee breaks. And you certainly won't want to listen to everyone else's weight problems. So give them a copy of this book, and soon even they won't be talking about losing weight. You can then all talk about the weather.

This kind of "food" definitely does not teach anyone about healthy eating. On the other hand, one can't overlook the convenience factor, which seems to be very important to boomers. I suppose given the choice, I'd rather see someone drink a Slim-Fast beverage or eat a Slim-Fast bar than skip a meal. However, I'd prefer to see this as the exception rather than the norm.

chapter 11

The High-Protein Diet Debate: What Happens Right After You Eat

My favorite animal is steak.

—Fran Lebowitz

Should you be a meat eater or a vegetarian? Or should you be somewhere in between? High-protein diets like the Atkins Diet, the Zone, and Protein Power have gotten more press time than advertising money could have bought. These programs are the major players in the high-protein-diets-are-good-for-you camp. Opposing these plans are those who believe a high-carbohydrate diet is better. Dr. Dean Ornish and Dr. John McDougall represent a more vegetarian approach to losing weight. Somewhere in between sits the USDA Food Guide Pyramid and the suggestions of the American Diabetes Association, the American Heart Association, and the American Dietetic Association. So who are you to believe?

People on a high-protein diet lose a lot of weight (if they can stick to the plan long enough). Yet people on a high-carbohydrate diet have similar results (if they, too, can stick to it). Guess what? Even those diet plans that sit in the middle of the two extremes can help you lose weight. Hmmm? Maybe there is no magic formula.

What the USDA Has to Say

Even the government is wondering if there's a magic formula. On February 24, 2000, the USDA brought together some of the most knowledgeable people in the nutrition field to participate in the "Great Nutrition Debate." They were there to determine who was right—the proponents of the high-protein diet or those who support the high-carbohydrate diet. With obesity continuing to rise, the government needs to figure out what's causing the problem and how it can be solved.

When Shirley Watkins, the Undersecretary for Food, Nutrition, and Consumer Services at the USDA, opened the conference that day, she shared a joke she'd recently heard:

> A man goes into his doctor's office, and there's a banana stuck in one ear, and a carrot stuck in the other one, and a cucumber up his nose. The man says, "Doctor, this is terrible. What's wrong with me?" The doctor simply said, "Well, first of all, you're not eating right."

So are we eating right? Each of the participants at the conference had a chance to speak, including Dr. Robert Atkins about his *Dr. Atkins New Diet Revolution,* Dr. Barry Sears for his *Zone Diet,* Dr. John McDougall for *McDougall's Right Foods Diet*, and Dr. Dean Ornish, author of *Eat More, Weigh Less.* After all the discussion, the conclusion was it's a matter of calories, not nutrients. If the American public ate fewer calories, whether they be high in protein or high in carbohydrates, they'd lose weight. No magic formula!

When you think about it, how can there be so many different diets purporting to be "the one," when all of them work some of the time? Better to ask three important questions:

- Is this diet safe?
- Can I maintain my new weight?
- Can I live with this approach the rest of my life?

If it's an approach that isn't healthy for you or can't be maintained indefinitely, then what's the value of spending part of your life doing it? You're setting yourself up for yo-yo dieting.

Part of the problem rests in the mind-set of a dieter. I've said it before, but I'll say it again: When you want to lose weight, you can't think you're going *on* a diet, only to get *off* of it in the future. The most extreme-type diets set people up for that mind-set, because what they ask of people is more than people can or are willing to do indefinitely. Keep in mind the three criteria I just listed for determining whether a diet is worthy of being followed.

The high-protein diet requires that you eliminate breads, pasta, rice, grains, milk, fruits, and pretty much everything else except meat, fat, and vegetables. On the other hand, the high-carbohydrate diets require that you include everything that the high-protein diets say to avoid, while having you drastically cut down on meat and fats. Fortunately, the high-carbohydrate diets encourage you to eat plenty of vegetables and fruits. The diets in the middle try to provide a balance between the two approaches.

It's important to remember that these diets have one thing in common—they're all low in calories. That, my dear reader, is really the answer to weight loss. Eat less + burn more through exercise = lose weight. "Badda bing, badda bang, badda boom." The final decision of what you eat is really yours. However, in order to make that decision, it's valuable for you to have a basic understanding of what your body does with the nutrients you feed it. Then you can make an educated choice.

What Happens to the Food Right After You Eat?

After you've eaten a mixed meal of carbohydrates, protein, and fat, your body goes to work. First, it must break down the food into smaller pieces and digest it, which is done in your stomach and intestines. The fats, proteins, and carbohydrates from your meal pass into your bloodstream as fatty acids, amino acids, and glucose, respectively. If you look at the following diagram, you should be able to follow the path of these nutrients. Take a little time to see where each of the nutrients is going after it's absorbed.

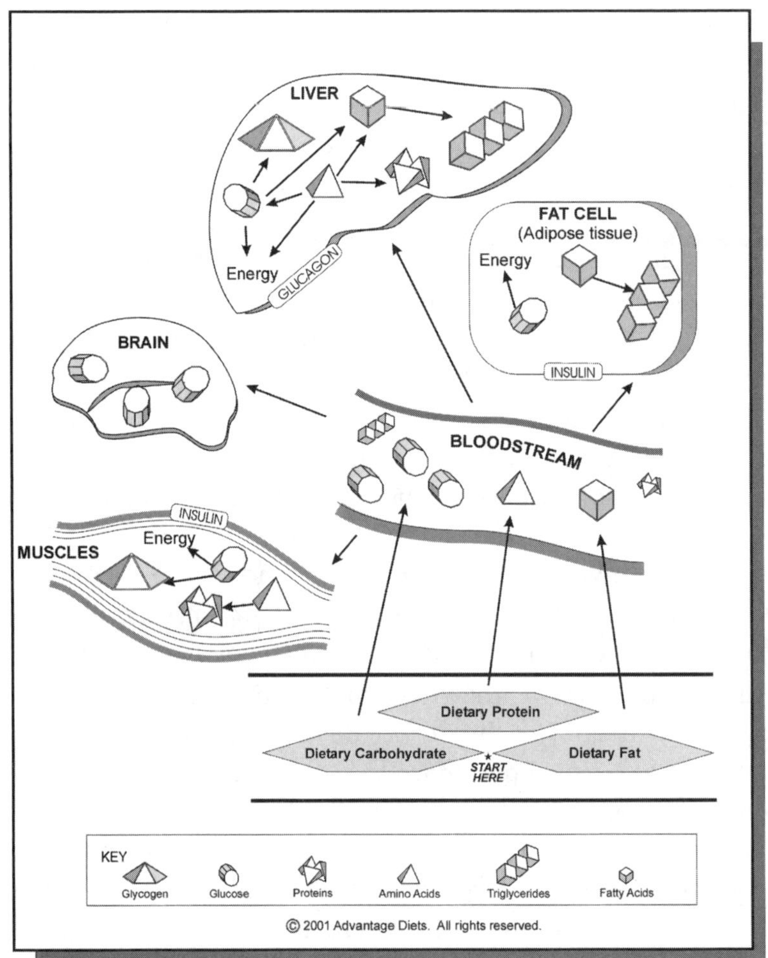

What happens to the food right after you eat.

When you eat something, your body's first objective is to use the nutrients in the food for any immediate needs. The rest is put into storage to ensure that there will be fuel available for later, when you're not eating.

The **fat** you eat in your diet is broken down into fatty acids. Some of these fatty acids go to your fat cells, to be stored as *triglycerides,* as you can see in the following figure. Your liver gets some of that fat as well, and stores it as triglycerides. When you've had a cholesterol test done by your doctor, you've probably had your triglycerides checked at the same time. It tells you how much fat is traveling around in your bloodstream.

The fatty acids that attach to the glycerol molecule are a direct reflection of your diet. If you've been eating a lot of saturated fat (such as from meat, butter, and so on), those fatty acids you see in the diagram are going to be predominately saturated. If, on the other hand, you've been eating a lot of monounsaturated fats (let's say from olive or canola oil) or polyunsaturated fats (from corn oil, safflower oil, and so forth), the fatty acid branches will reflect those fats. If we were to take a sample of your fat tissue, we'd be able to see what kind of diet you've been eating.

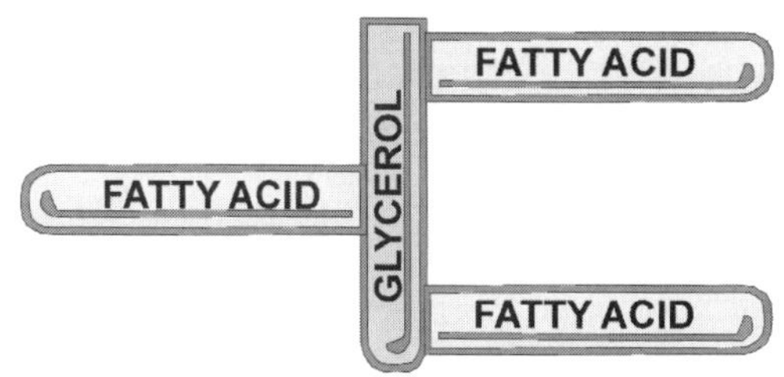

A triglyceride is a glycerol backbone with three ("tri") fatty acids attached.

What happens to the **proteins** you eat? After being digested in your intestine, they're absorbed as *amino acids,* which go to your muscles and liver. Once in your liver, the amino acid's destiny is determined by what proteins the body needs, such as hormones, enzymes, secretions, and so on. The amino acids may be passed back out to the bloodstream to be picked up by the muscles and other tissues to be used locally. They may even be used for energy. Keep this last point in mind when I tell you about energy sources on a high-protein diet.

Last, the **carbohydrates,** which have been broken down into *glucose* molecules, enter your bloodstream, raising your blood sugar level. Your liver, muscle, brain, fat cells, and other tissues pick up the glucose from your blood, until your blood sugar level returns to normal. When glucose enters your liver, it may be used immediately for energy or converted into *glycogen* (a compact storage form of glucose). It will be used later when you're not eating, to maintain a normal level of glucose in your blood.

From the figure on the preceding page you can see that glucose enters your muscle cells at the same time it's going to your liver, brain, and fat cells. It is first used for energy in your muscles; after that need has been satisfied, the extra in your muscles is converted into glycogen for storage. When your blood sugar gets low, your liver provides glucose to the blood. The glycogen that's stored in your muscles has no way to get back out into your bloodstream. So it remains there for use as energy for the muscles.

Your liver can only hold so much glycogen. When there's more glucose than your liver can store as glycogen or can use for immediate energy needs, the liver converts the excess to fat. This is dropped into your bloodstream as triglycerides and then picked up by your fat cells. You can see, then, how a diet high in calories and carbohydrates encourages the production of triglycerides when the liver can't store it all as glycogen. (When you have your blood tested and get a triglyceride count, some of those triglycerides traveling around your blood may have been excess glucose that your liver converted and is now on its way to your fat cells.) The same fate holds true for excess protein, which is eventually converted to fat, as well. Let me emphasize that point—**excess carbohydrates and excess proteins become fat. There they join the excess fat in your fat cells and add to your weight.** That's truly the bottom line when it comes to being overweight—too much of anything isn't a good thing.

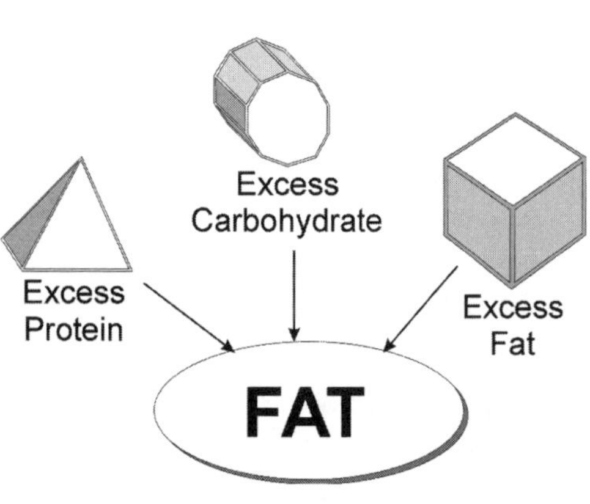

The fate of the nutrients.

With a Little Help

Did you notice the word *insulin* on the fat cell and muscle cell in the first figure? Insulin is a hormone made in the pancreas that acts as a key to open the doors of your cells, helping nutrients enter their target cell locations. But notice that the liver and the brain don't require insulin to absorb glucose. Because the brain's major energy source is glucose, it would be very inefficient for it to have to depend upon insulin to be around to get its food. As you will soon see, if you're on a high-protein diet, there isn't as much glucose around to feed the brain and so it has to depend upon another energy source: fat.

The amount of glucose that's circulating in the blood is the major determinant of how much insulin is released from the pancreas. If you eat a lot of sugar at one time, which will be quickly absorbed, your pancreas needs to respond just as quickly with insulin. Your body doesn't really like having a high blood sugar—so when the amount of glucose in your blood spikes, so does the amount of insulin. After enough glucose has been removed from your bloodstream, insulin secretion is suppressed.

What If Your Meal Is Mostly Protein?

Whenever your meal is mostly proteins, *glucagon,* another hormone, is released from the pancreas. This signals the liver to deposit some of its stored glucose into the bloodstream. Glucagon has an opposite mission from insulin—if the glucose level in your bloodstream is too low, it tries to raise it. The more carbohydrates you eat with the protein in your meal, the less glucagon has to be secreted, allowing the liver to save its glucose for later when you're not eating.

I hope you're with me so far. Because now it gets interesting. What do you think happens to all the protein you eat on a high-protein diet? Not all of it goes into your muscles. Some of it's absorbed by your liver. The likelihood is that your liver won't need all those amino acids for making the various proteins for your body, so it has to do something with the excess.

Keeping in mind that maintaining a normal blood sugar requires glucose, and that the meal you just had was mostly protein, your liver is going to have to get to work. First, it converts some of the excess amino acids into glucose. In the process of converting protein to glucose, your liver has to remove the nitrogen from the amino acid. That nitrogen must be eliminated from your body. Nitrogen cannot freely float around in your bloodstream—it's toxic. So your liver packages it up as *urea.* Urea is then excreted in your urine. (Have you ever noticed that when you eat a lot of protein, you urinate more? This is part of the reason. The body has to use fluids to carry the urea out.) Sounds simple enough, except that you're making your kidneys work overtime to get rid of that excess urea. It can be taxing on the kidneys, something we don't need as we get older. It's bad enough that your kidneys are aging naturally, where they don't filter quite as efficiently as they used to. I certainly don't see any reason to rush the process by stressing them with what we eat. In addition, if you don't increase your fluid intake, you can become dehydrated.

Another problem with a high-protein diet and its effect on your kidneys is that all that urea makes your urine more acidic. This acidic environment encourages the formation of kidney stones (especially for those who are prone to making stones). When urea is excreted, it takes some calcium with it. This calcium can join up with some oxalates or phosphates and form a stone. Where do you think that calcium came from? It's pulled out of your bones. Next thing you know you could be suffering from osteoporosis (a weakening of the bones). This isn't to imply that a high-protein diet is going to cause all this to happen or happen right away. You just have a higher chance that it could.

After your liver has converted the excess amino acids into glucose, it sends the glucose out into your bloodstream to try to maintain a normal blood sugar. In most cases, there isn't enough excess protein to both supply the blood with glucose and maintain adequate glycogen stores.

Not to worry. Your body has a backup method to save the day. It calls on your fat cells to give up some of their fat to use for energy.

chapter 12

The High-Protein Diet Debate: What Happens Between Meals

Red meat is not bad for you. Now blue-green meat, that's bad for you!

—Tommy Smothers

Your blood sugar is going to drop between meals unless your body can come up with some glucose. Only your liver can provide glucose to the bloodstream. Depending on whether you've been eating balanced meals or high-protein meals, the process is different. Let's look at where the energy is going to come from.

When You Eat a Balanced Diet

The process of supplying energy to the body is really a lot like the reverse of what happened when your body stored the nutrients away after you ate. Look at the following figure as I share some of the details with you. Your blood sugar is dropping and various parts of your body respond. Your liver gives up some of its glycogen stores in the form of glucose. Your muscles contribute some amino acids, and your fat cells give up some triglycerides; both go to the liver to be converted to glucose. The idea is to keep the storehouse of glycogen in your liver well stocked, while your liver is supplying some of its glucose to your bloodstream. This is easy to accomplish when you eat a balanced diet with sufficient protein and carbohydrates.

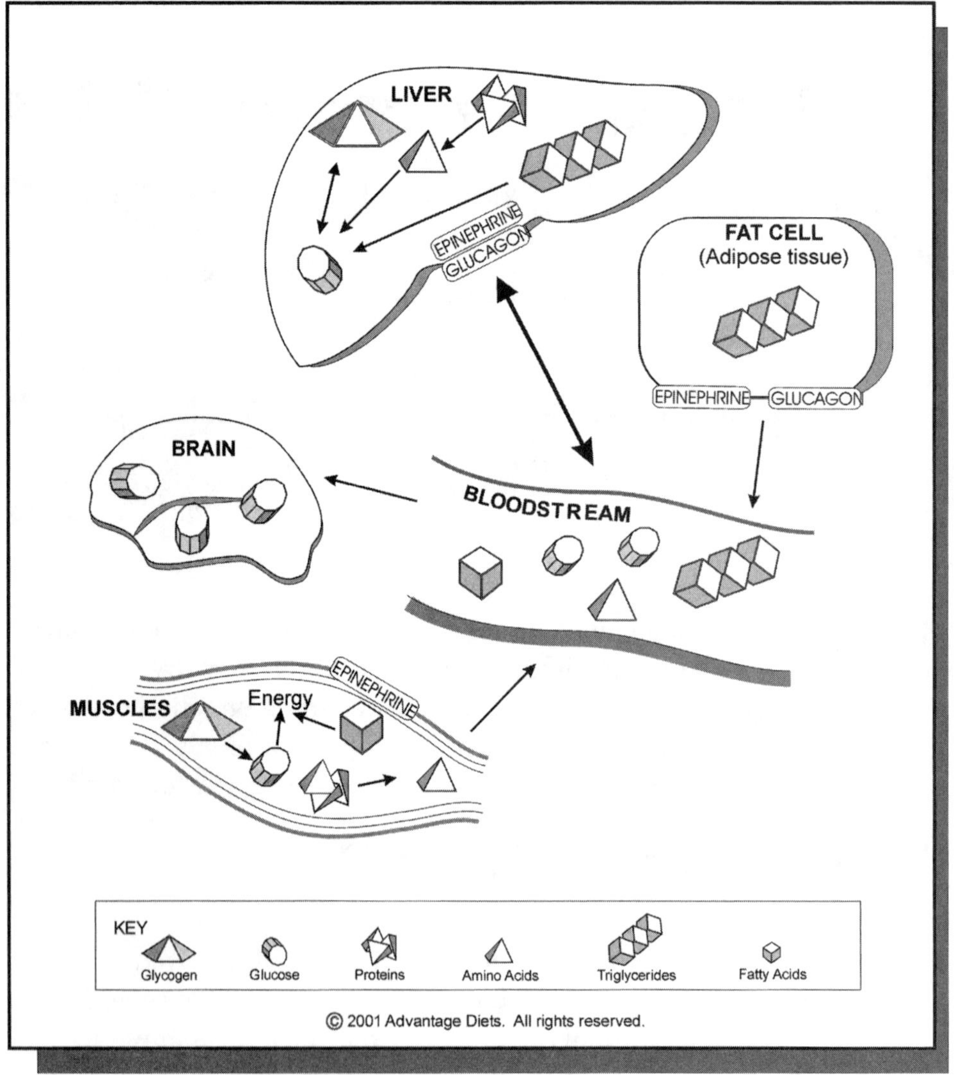

Energy sources on a balanced diet.

When You Eat a High-Protein Diet

Before I share with you what happens when you've been eating a high-protein diet, I'd like to give you an idea of what's meant by a high-protein diet. The two major diet plans, available in book form, are *The Zone*, by Barry Sears, Ph.D., and *Dr. Atkins New Diet Revolution*, by Dr. Robert C. Atkins. Sears proposes a 40–30–30 mix of nutrients to "stay in the zone," where he says you shouldn't have spikes of insulin. Those numbers represent 40 percent of calories from carbohydrates, 30 percent from protein, and 30 percent from fat. In contrast, the Atkins diet is approximately 10–30–60, with 10 percent of calories from carbohydrates, 30 percent from protein, and a whopping 60 percent from fat (with no restrictions on saturated fat, which can lead to increased blood cholesterol and heart disease). These percentage allocations are in stark contrast to the current recommendations from the American Heart Association, the American Dietetic Association, and the United States Department of Agriculture (Food Guide Pyramid). These organizations recommend 50 to 55 percent of calories from carbohydrates, 15 to 20 percent from protein, and less than 30 percent from fat.

On a high-protein diet, the glycogen stores in your liver could be depleted or in short supply. Now where's the energy going to come from, and what's going to feed your brain? Remember, it's waiting for its glucose meal. Even though your muscles and fat cells are donating amino acids and fatty acids to your liver, your liver doesn't have enough time to convert these to enough glucose to raise the blood sugar sufficiently. If it had the glycogen stores it normally has with a balanced diet, there would be immediate glucose. Instead, the fat from your fat cells is converted to *ketones* in your liver. It's a fairly rapid process, and your body can use ketones for energy if it has to. Even your brain will use ketones if glucose isn't available. You can see what happens in the following figure. Now instead of having your bloodstream teeming with glucose, it's teeming with ketones.

Anyone who's been on a high-protein diet knows the routine. You measure your urine for ketones using a "lipolysis test strip." If you have enough ketones in your urine, the paper should change color. For those of you who've tried this diet, you know the thrill of seeing the paper turn a deep purple color. It means that your fat cells are making a big donation to the energy equation. And because losing weight means losing fat, it seems like you're accomplishing the feat.

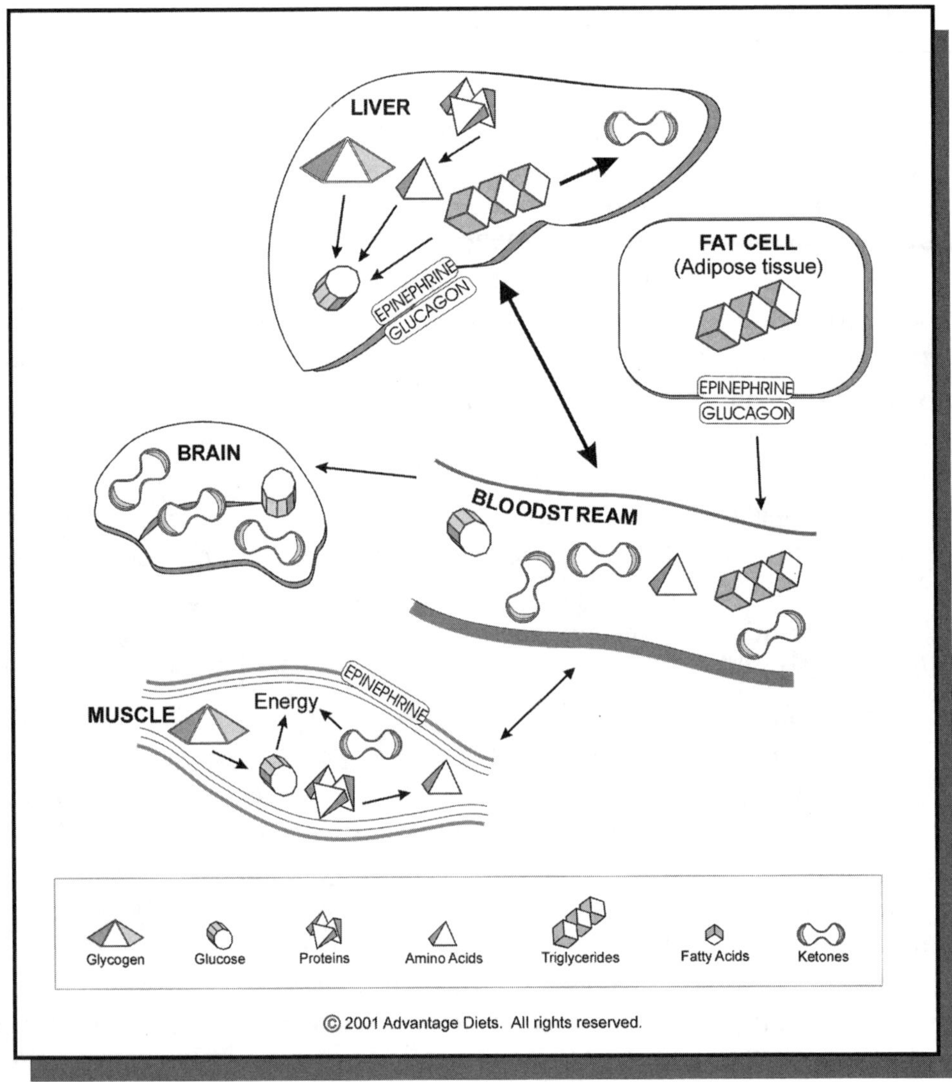

Energy sources on a high-protein diet.

The Good and the Bad of It

Don't jump on the high-protein diet bandwagon just yet. Remember what I told you in the last chapter, that too much protein can affect your kidneys and your bones. That would give me cause to pause. Also, because so many foods are eliminated from the diet, there should be a concern for not getting an adequate amount of nutrients. And there's no way, as I have shared with you, that eating all the saturated fat you get on a high-protein diet can be healthy for you. One minor side effect of the diet, which you may or may not be aware of, is that you could have bad breath—the result of all those ketones in your blood. Another problem is constipation, because the diet is so low in fiber.

With all that said, many people who've tried the high-protein diets say they're pleased with the weight loss, but eventually get bored with eating just meat. They miss a slice of bread once in a while, or a baked potato. One positive aspect to reducing the amount of carbohydrates in the diet is that it does get people to give up eating simple sugars. I think that when we eat a lot of sugar, we stimulate the need for more. I have found the same to be true for fat. When people start eating a lower-fat diet, they find it hard going back to eating a lot of fat. It just tastes too greasy. I can't drink whole milk anymore. It's like drinking a cup of cream.

Another plus to the higher protein intake is its ability to satisfy your appetite. It's partly due to the fact that it takes protein longer to digest. In addition, the increased amount of fat in a high-protein diet helps to delay the stomach from emptying. However, the major reason that protein works so well is it doesn't cause a spike in insulin as too many carbohydrates at one time can do. A spike in insulin can cause a too-rapid drop in blood sugar. This, in turn, can cause you to feel hungry and fatigued. The next thing you know, you need to eat again.

You Might Be Insulin Resistant

Another problem for overweight people that involves insulin is a condition called *insulin resistance.* When you eat a great deal of carbohydrates, your pancreas is forced to supply a lot of insulin. However, the cells of overweight people seem to resist the action of insulin. It's as if they've hung out a "do not disturb" sign, causing the glucose in the bloodstream to swim on by. This is especially true for muscle cells. The pancreas then figures it needs to provide more insulin to get the blood sugar under control, which just aggravates the problem. It doesn't matter. The cells are just not answering the call.

The excess insulin can lead to a condition called *hyperinsulinemia,* which is a risk factor (though not necessarily a cause) for the development of

Type 2 diabetes (non-insulin-dependent), hypertension, and cardiovascular disease (due to increased levels of triglycerides in the blood and lower levels of HDL, the "good" cholesterol).

So it's understandable why people think that a high-protein diet is the answer. But with all the side effects of high-protein, I think a more balanced diet makes sense. By combining carbohydrates and proteins in one meal, the carbohydrates are not digested and absorbed as rapidly. The proteins are able to dampen the effect, keeping the glucose level and, in turn, the insulin level, in the blood from spiking. If you add exercise to your routine, you make the cells more sensitive to the insulin so they'll respond more quickly.

I believe that a big part of the problem is eating far too many simple carbohydrates—in other words, sugar in one form or another. Sometimes you don't even know you're eating it because many fat-free products use sugar to replace the fat. People assume it's healthier for them because it's fat-free. We had that message drummed into our heads in the 1980s that we should be eating as much "fat free" as possible. But all that sugar can be causing problems for those with insulin resistance. Some believe that instead of increasing the protein in the diet, it's better to emphasize complex carbohydrates and increase the amount of fat slightly (the monounsaturated variety found in olive and canola oils). It has a neutral effect on insulin secretion. And if it's the healthy kind of fat, it shouldn't affect your blood cholesterol in a negative way. Only time will tell what future studies will reveal to us about the right percentages for each nutrient. Until then, moderation makes the most sense.

> *Once a vampire has tasted blood, you'll never make him a vegetarian.*
>
> —*Paul W. Lawrence*

There is one other downside to a high-protein diet. Eating a goodly amount of protein as your energy source is an expensive way to go. Let's say you buy 1 pound of steak for $4.99 and a 1-pound loaf of bread for $1.99. After your body has taken the protein it needs from the steak, the excess will be used for energy. Keep in mind that the bread also provides energy. Comparing the cost of your energy, having it from the steak is costing you $3.00 more per pound than the energy from the bread. I can think of better ways to spend my money.

part 3

Quick, Get Me Out of This Mess

Everyone has his or her own reason for losing weight. One of the reasons I'd like you to consider is that you can reduce your risk for some of the major killers—heart disease, diabetes, and cancer. Weight is such a strong factor with these diseases that for you not to take off the pounds is quite possibly signing your own death warrant.

More important is how you're going to get the weight off—for good. Because of my background in personality typing, I've found that the approach you should take depends on your type. As you read the following chapters, you'll not only learn what part of your personality is involved in determining the weight-loss approach, but which plans would be right for you.

chapter 13

Break a Habit—Make a Habit

I used to say, "I sure hope things will change." Then I learned that the only way things are going to change for me is when I change.

—Jim Rohn

When you saw the title of this chapter, were you tempted to skip this subject, hoping to avoid having to admit to some of your not-so-healthy habits? Don't be ashamed. Everyone has some habits they'd love to get rid of, but seem to be holding onto, much like the cartoon character Linus, who drags his blanket with him wherever he goes. Baby boomers have had plenty of years of practice.

Worthless Willpower

Don't think it's a lack of willpower that's holding you back from changing. In fact, I think the use of willpower is the wrong approach, considering you're trying to change a habit for good. If you're planning to use willpower the rest of your life, you're going to be one exhausted and emotionally drained person. Think about a time when you had to use willpower to avoid doing something or, conversely, to do something. How did you feel? Deprived? Annoyed? How long did those efforts last? It's a rare person who has changed a habit permanently using willpower.

I believe that people who want to lose weight end up yo-yo dieting for two reasons. Either they're using willpower to avoid eating certain foods and find they can't maintain that vigilance, or the method they're using to lose weight isn't comfortable for them, so it isn't an approach they can follow the rest of their lives. If they've successfully lost weight, they say to themselves, "I'm glad that's over"—and then go back to the habits that got them overweight in the first place. I can't say it enough times, no one should ever "go on a diet."

> To go *on* a diet means eventually going *off* a diet. The idea is to discover an effective way to eat that doesn't look, feel, or taste like a diet.

People use willpower as a way of avoiding facing up to the reason for or cause of the bad habit. Instead, they impose something external that seems healthier (for example, a new diet plan); then they grit their teeth to make it work. I suppose they figure that if they use willpower long enough, the new behavior they're practicing will replace the bad habit and become their new healthy habit. Sometimes that works. However, more often than not, their willpower crumbles and they revert to the old habit, feeling like a failure. Moreover, they still haven't faced up to what caused the bad habit.

Jane, an older baby boomer, was born shortly after the end of World War II. Her parents, having had to scrape by during the war, now could afford to put more food on the table, and give treats besides. If Jane didn't eat everything on her plate, she was soundly reminded of how bad everything was during the war or how children were starving overseas. She inevitably developed "clean-the-plate" syndrome—not an easy habit to break. Now she's an adult and yet she's still cleaning her plate. Deciding it's time to lose weight, she goes on a diet, using whatever willpower she can muster to leave something on her plate. Everything is going fine until one day something happens in her life that's so stressful her willpower no longer works. Jane doesn't care what the diet says; she eats everything on her plate. There—now she feels like her old self again, somehow figuring that her old self can handle this stress better than this make-believe person she seems to have become.

Do you see the problem here? Jane hadn't dealt with the reason why she learned to clean her plate. She didn't think about the fact that the times had changed. There was no longer the we-didn't-have-it-and-now-we-do influence. At the end of the chapter, you'll learn more about what it means to let go of an old image.

Born with a Clean Slate

Do you realize that the day you were born you had no habits? You were a clean slate. Over the years, you've written on that slate. Because we're talking about habits, you may wonder how you can erase that slate so you can start fresh. I wouldn't want to see you do that. Not all of your habits are unhealthy ones, so let's not, as the saying goes, "throw the baby out with the bath water."

Some habits make life easier. Can you imagine having to stop and think through every step of tying your shoelaces? Step 1: Pull the laces up tight. Step 2: Cross the right lace over the left lace. Step 3: Pass the right lace under the left lace. And so on. Ugh! The idea of dealing with all aspects of life this way is gruesome. Nobody would ever get anything accomplished. So there is something to be said about having habits—healthy ones, that is.

Before we can get to the root of a habit, we need to become aware of it. Awareness, though, is just the first step. What's interesting, and almost embarrassing to admit, is that we're often aware of a habit, realize it isn't good for us, but continue to do it anyway. Have you ever stopped to ask yourself "why am I doing this or that?" For example, "Why am I eating the whole pint container of Häagen-Dazs ice cream, when I'm not even hungry?" Not taking a moment to ponder may be part of the problem.

I have an exercise for you to do. Take a piece of paper and title it "My Top Ten List of Unhealthy Habits." List major and minor habits. Think of them in terms of how they're holding you back from achieving your weight-loss goals. If you can't come up with 10, check the end of this chapter for some ideas. No peeking now! Try making your own list first. After each habit, state why you think you have that habit, and include the influences that help you maintain it. Then, on a scale of 1 to 5 (1 being easy to change and 5 being hard to change), rate how easy or hard you think it would be to change each habit. For example, "I eat a dish of ice cream every night. That's because my husband insists I join him when he has some. In order not to get into an argument with him, I eat it to keep the peace. I'd rank this a 5 because it's not just me involved in the process of changing the habit."

Try this: Every time you start to eat, ask yourself, (1) "Why am I eating?" and (2) "Why am I eating this?" It should be interesting to watch yourself and see how many reasons (often known as excuses) you give.

Another idea is to create a table with three columns with the headings: "What's the situation?" "How do I normally handle it?" and "What's a better way?" For example, the *situation* is that I skipped breakfast because I didn't have time to make it and was ravenous by midmorning. *Normally,* I'll grab something out of the vending machine. A *better way* would be to make a breakfast sandwich (for example, toasted whole-wheat English muffin topped with scrambled egg, sliced apple, and a sprinkle of cinnamon) the night before and take it to work with me.

You might be trying to mask a bad habit with what appears to be a healthier habit—by using willpower. The woman in the preceding ice cream example decided that the way to fix her problem was to commit to never eating ice cream again. She'd just sit there with her husband and have a cup of tea. She figured that she was replacing an unhealthy habit with a healthy one. How long do you think her ultimatum lasted? Just until she slipped and had a bite of ice cream. After that, all she could think about was how she had failed.

This situation is very common. People put themselves into a "no choice" situation, imposing restrictions that they think will save them from themselves. It's a you-can-never-have-this-again mentality. Unless your doctor has told you not to eat something, or you're allergic to a particular food, why eliminate something forever? Part of losing weight and maintaining a healthy body is establishing a healthy relationship with food.

As baby boomers, we've come to expect myriad choices in everything related to our lives. Back when Henry Ford brought out the Model T, a person could get one model in any color—as long as it was black! Look at the automotive industry today. There are so many different models, and a Crayola box of colors from which to choose. The boomer generation, in fact, has grown up expecting the opportunity to choose from many alternatives. With that in mind, why would you be satisfied being told that there's only one way to lose weight, and good luck if it's not a way that works for you? You're given no choice. That's why I've provided a number of different approaches in this book to allow you the freedom to make the choice. You know yourself better than I do.

Getting to the Root of the Habit

Becoming aware of a problem is not enough. You need to explore why you have a particular unhealthy habit. By discovering the reasons behind an unhealthy habit, you can let go of and bury it. Otherwise, it may be just a matter of time before it rears its ugly head again. From your Top Ten list, ask yourself if any of those unhealthy habits serve any purpose in your life. If they do, then you need to deal with them directly. If they don't, get out the shovel and bury them.

When you're trying to figure out why you have particular habits, be careful that you don't defend them with some lame excuses. Blaming someone or something outside of you won't work. Have you ever noticed that when you point your finger, more of your fingers are aimed back at yourself than at your target? (Try it and you'll see.) Hmmmm! Something interesting to think about.

Unfortunately, habits are often rooted in emotions. Stressed out? Bored? Overwhelmed? Angry? Afraid? How do you react to these emotions? Many react by eating. When you were younger, were you given a cookie or a piece of candy to make things all better? Too many of us think, *why not now?*

The findings from the American Dietetic Association's nationwide public opinion survey, "Nutrition and You: Trends 2002," shed a little light on how important nutrition and physical activity are to adults today. It also showed how likely they may be to change their habits.

The survey showed that 38 percent of Americans fall into the "I'm Already Doing It" category (to which I say, keep up the good work!), 30 percent are in the "I Know I Should, But" category (there's hope here yet!), and the remaining 32 percent say "Don't Bother Me" (whoops!).

Re-Imaging

As you read this section, you may find it strange that I suggest there be an end before a beginning. Most people wanting to lose weight assume that the weight-loss process starts with a beginning. Yet before you can see yourself as lean and fit, you need to let go of the present image you have of yourself; this is the ***ending.*** You can't lose weight if you continue to see yourself as a fat person trying to become thin.

The first step is to get rid of your old identity. I know you're probably saying that that's impossible. You see yourself every day in the mirror. What I'm suggesting is performing a ritual of sorts; we'll call it a "good-riddance ceremony." Take a recent picture of yourself. Get a cookie tin or frying pan that can withstand some flames. Create a ceremonial environment—maybe some candles and soft music. Place the picture in the heat-resistant container. As you light a match to it, say good-bye to this body you want to change. Let go of all the mental baggage that you've been carrying with you regarding your weight. Watch the photo as it burns to ashes. From now on, every time you start thinking about yourself as a heavy person, remember the photo-burning ceremony. You're moving forward.

After you have experienced an end, you can then make the transition to wherever you want to go. However, before you enter the new beginning phase, you may go through a period that feels awkward to you. I like to refer to it as the ***interim*** phase. You will be experimenting to find ways of losing weight that are comfortable to follow for a lifetime.

At times, you can be strongly motivated to do something. At other times, become anxious that the motivation seems to be flagging. You might even find some old unhealthy habits coming back. Methods you're trying might not be working. The idea is to go with the flow and don't give up. If viewed correctly, this can be a most exciting time because finally something is being done. The interim phase isn't necessarily a straight line from the ending to the new beginning. There may be many turns and bumps in the road before it becomes clear where this is all headed.

The last phase, the ***new beginning,*** is when you feel you have eating, exercising, and handling stress under control. You don't have to have reached your goal weight to say you are now in the new beginning phase. However, it may take some time to get there. The feeling you have about yourself and what you're doing will let you know you've arrived.

Achieving your goal weight will take time, but having established the route you'll take to get there is a vital an element to your success. After you feel you've created some healthy habits, celebrate with an "arrival ceremony" (just as you had a good-riddance ceremony). Most people tend to think ceremonies must be accompanied by food. That's not what I had in mind. I think going out and buying some new clothes would be a good start. Then, collect all your "big" clothes and give them to your local thrift shop. Do something festive while wearing your new clothes, showing off how far you've come. If you have a great way to celebrate, let me know and I'll share it with others.

Taking Control

Baby boomers are actually a fairly independent lot. We definitely had more freedoms growing up than our parents did. Many of us patiently waited until the freedoms were given to us. Others, known collectively as the hippie generation, decided for themselves that it was time—and took control.

To feel you can successfully change your habits, you need to believe that you are in control of your habits—rather than the other way around. To give you an idea of what I mean, when you're watching television, who has custody of the remote control? If it's not you, would you like to have it occasionally? If so, then you know the feeling of not being in control, not being able to decide what channel to watch or what volume is right.

Unhealthy habits can be changed! Don't let them control your life, when you have the power to control them. Even though you created those habits, it can sometimes feel like it's you against them. To give those habits the upper hand is to succumb to them rather than fight them. If you *need* those habits, they've won. If you *want* those habits, then you have the freedom to choose. Look at the Top Ten list again and decide whether there's a need or a want with each of them. If it's a need, you might think about seeking professional help—because the habit may be an addiction.

Stages of Change

Few people are able to just say "I'm going to lose weight" and then go do it. More often than not, it's a gradual warming up to the idea. Read about the different stages and determine at which level you think you are. It will make a difference in how successful you can be. Starting when you're not ready doesn't bode well for success.

"Who, me, have a problem?" At this stage, a person can't even see that he or she has a problem. That's why people who've been told by a loved one to lose weight probably won't be successful—it wasn't even their idea. Of course, it's possible for one to deny that there is a problem or place the blame elsewhere. ("It's my genes." "My mother forced me to clean my plate and now I can't break the habit.") Are you at this stage?

"Don't rush me. I'm thinking about it." At this stage, people are willing to admit that they're overweight, wonder what caused it, and will begin to think about how to fix it. Getting started will often be challenging, because people don't want to risk failing. They'll do a great deal of thinking about it, but seem to be procrastinating about taking any action. Are you at this stage?

"Okay. I'm looking into it." At this stage, one is getting closer to actually doing something. Some people start to make their intent public. Others will keep it to themselves until they're ready to actually take action. Thoughts of how to go about losing weight start to surface. I would say that because you're reading this book, you're in the "Okay. I'm looking into it" stage. Are you?

"Let the games begin. I'm charged up and ready to go." This is the exciting stage. It's finally time to do something. Of course, it will take time and energy. This is the step at which you must "break habits." You'll be experiencing many changes, especially with regard to your self-image and the way people perceive you. Don't let others defeat your good intentions because they can't handle the changes you'll be experiencing.

"Just keep on keepin' on." This may be the most important stage—and maybe the most difficult. It will take a great deal of commitment on your part, a continued heightened awareness of what you're doing, and a realization that none of this can happen overnight. However, you'll probably find this stage easier than you've experienced on other diets, because you lost weight in a way that was comfortable for you. Now is the time you're continuing the pattern you've established.

"It's working. It's really working." At this stage you should no longer have to police yourself, consciously watching your every move and worrying about some possible misstep. What you've learned should have become part of you. Because you never "went *on* a diet," as discussed earlier, you're not at this stage "going *off* a diet." You're living life normally as a fit person.

Unhealthy habits include the following:

- I tend to overcommit myself.
- I eat a lot of junk food because it is cheap and easy.
- I tend to set unrealistic goals for myself.
- I eat even when I'm not hungry.
- I eat food because it's there.
- I eat when I'm bored, tired, or depressed.
- I lead too sedentary a life.
- Exercise is always last on the list of things to do.
- I make excuses for all of the above.

chapter 14

The Diet That Isn't a Diet

It's so hard when I have to, and so easy when I want to.

—Sondra Anice Barnes

"Jennifer, you've just got to try this new diet I'm on," exclaimed Linda. "After all the yo-yo dieting I've done over the years, I think I've finally found the right one. I'm successfully losing weight." Because Linda was so thrilled with her accomplishment, she had to share the news with her friend. Jennifer had recently told Linda that she promised herself that this was the year to get into shape. Jennifer had had her weight-loss successes, but most were short-lived. The pounds she'd lose seemed to have a homing instinct—they kept coming back. The idea that someone had finally discovered the right diet energized her to try again. After several months, though, she found she wasn't having the success that her friend boasted about. She tried using willpower, and found it didn't help. So she gave up and once again believed that she was a failure at dieting.

Then there's Adam, who'd been talking about losing weight for a very long time but just couldn't seem to get started. He finally decided one Saturday that he would begin, only to remember that he was supposed to go to a dinner party that night. How could he possibly insult his hostess by turning down her delicious meal? So he promised himself that his diet would start the following Monday morning. It seems as if his boss had other plans for him, though, dumping a huge load of work on his desk along with an impending deadline to finish it. Adam felt he didn't have the time, space, or mental capacity to devote to changing his eating habits while trying to get the job done for his boss.

Marianne's challenge wasn't one of getting started on a diet, but of staying on track. She's a mother of two, a preschooler and a second-grader. While wanting to be sure they ate well, she didn't want to deny them treats. The problem with having those treats in the house is that Marianne found it very difficult to resist indulging in them herself. They seemed to constantly call out to her, saying "eat us, eat us." Before she knew it, she'd respond to their call. They were gone—and guilt had taken their place.

These are just a few of my clients' stories about their struggles with losing weight. Do any of them sound familiar? As you can see, you're not alone. In fact, it seems to be a problem for an estimated 64 percent of Americans who are overweight or obese. Every year billions of dollars are spent on diet pills, diet foods, exercise equipment, videos, counseling, health clubs, and so on. How many diets have you been on, only to be frustrated and upset when you found out that that one didn't work for you either? Do you ever wonder why all your hard work doesn't seem to produce significant or lasting results? Or wonder why you can't even get started? You might tend to unfairly blame yourself, thinking that you're a failure.

> *You always pass failure on the way to success.*
>
> —*Mickey Rooney*

"I'm a Failure, So Why Try?"

We have an obesity epidemic facing our nation. *What could have caused it?* That question is fairly easy to answer—we've become a very sedentary society, we eat too many high-fat foods, and we're not careful about how much we eat. According to the 2000 U.S. census, the highest rate of overweight and obesity occurred in the boomer age bracket. You can't even use the excuse that as people get older, they tend to get fatter. The percentage of those in the 65 years and over group who are overweight or obese is about 10 percent lower than the boomer group.

What can you do to stop it? That question is a little harder to answer. The most obvious approach would be to take a good look at *what* and *how much* you're eating—that may have to change. No one would debate the issue that too many calories eaten and not enough burned off puts weight on. So exercise also has to be included. However, and more importantly, it would be good to look at *how* you're going to change. When people don't get the results they were hoping for from a diet, I like to say, "You didn't fail. The plan failed you." **Which just means that if you could find the "right" way, it should be easy.**

Think back on the various diets you've tried. What made you try them in the first place? Are you like Jennifer, who's willing to try a diet a friend had success on, even though it doesn't mean that it's well suited for her? Of course, your friend's enthusiasm may be too strong to ignore. Maybe the diet plan appeared easy, where all you had to do was pop a pill? Yet, there is no way you'll have permanent weight loss popping pills because you didn't change any of the lifestyle habits that caused you to gain weight in the first place.

Why do you think the diets you've tried haven't worked? From my experience, I believe I have the answer. **You need to follow a plan that's comfortable for who you are.**

So Who Are You?

Two facets of your personality can strongly influence the type of diet plan that would work best for you. As I describe the two facets of how you live your life, think of which one seems the most like you. Even though you find similarities to yourself in both descriptions, it's the one that comes closest that's important. The first description will be that of what I call the "Planner"—the second one I call the "Ad-libber."

Making a decision. If you're a Planner, you tend to speak with a sense of authority. You believe in standards and rules that, when followed, make life easier. Whether someone wants it or not, you're not afraid to give advice. Most of the time that advice is based on having done your homework, so you can feel confident in what you say and the decisions you make. However, that's not to say that your homework is complete, because you're often in a hurry to get it done and out of the way. In order to make a decision, you collect whatever information seems necessary, narrow down the possibilities, and then decide quickly. After you've made a decision, you may ignore new facts, because those details might just cloud the issue. You're normally not a second-guesser.

By comparison, if you're an Ad-libber, the more possibilities there are the better. You figure if one fact doesn't apply, maybe another will. You don't want to be tied down to one fact, one approach, one way. You don't know for sure if it's the right way until it's been tested and tried. Because you really enjoy the adventure of exploring and trying new ways, it's okay if something isn't the standard approach. As for second-guessing, you do a lot of that. Fearing you may not have enough information, you may question the decisions you've made, and then go back and try to get more information. Keeping your options open is your byword. While the Planners are saying "that's final," Ad-libbers are saying "don't hold me to that."

Well, which way do you lean at this point? Planner? Ad-libber?

Keeping a date. You know you're a Planner by the day-timer you've got tucked under your arm. From your perspective, life goes so much more smoothly when you have it all scheduled. When you return home or to work, recently made dates will be dutifully copied onto your main calendar. You tend to be on time for appointments and meetings. By being scheduled, there are no surprises. However, when you appear frazzled, others know things didn't work out quite as you planned.

You Ad-libbers are the just the opposite. Keeping a calendar is much too restrictive. It means that after you've scheduled something, you feel boxed in by it. You prefer to keep your options open. There may be some last-minute opportunities you'd miss if your life were too scheduled. Whereas Planners are schedule-type people, you Ad-libbers are spontaneous-type people. You find adapting to a new event much easier than do Planners. Maybe that's because you tend to be more flexible.

Okay, how are you doing? Are you going with Planner or Ad-libber?

Endings versus beginnings. The best time for you Planners is when a project is completed. You can be persistent during the process, but closure is most important for you—especially a quick closure. That way, when the project is done you can move on to the next one. It's even better if you were able to complete the project on time. Remember, there's a schedule to keep. The fun part is planning and tracking the project, watching it come closer and closer to completion. This approach allows you a sense of control over what you're doing. It's better not to leave anything to chance.

On the other hand, you Ad-libbers love to start projects, but are less concerned about getting them done. If something is over too quickly, that means the experience ends. That's fine, if things aren't going well. But when you're having fun, why end it? With this attitude, projects can take many different turns along the way, which is great because you Ad-libbers like variety. That's what makes life interesting to you. One of the hallmark traits of an Ad-libber is using last-minute pressure to get a job done. That tension seems to spur you on to completion. Because the process tends to capture your attention, it's fine if the project continues indefinitely. You're able to just go with the flow.

So let's see how you're doing. Do you think you're a Planner or an Ad-libber?

Order and chaos. You Planners thrive on planning. It gives order to your life. You know what's expected of you and what you expect from others. Do you make lists? If so, you may be a Planner. It could be a to-do list, a list of where things are stored, or a list of errands that you need to run. Some of those lists may be so organized that the items on it are prioritized—which one is to be done first, second, and so on. The greatest thrill, if you're a Planner, is to draw a line through a completed item or put a checkmark next to it. You Planners want everything organized so that, whenever you're looking for something, it's easier to find. Filing cabinets and organizer boxes were made for you. There's logic to the way you organize.

You Ad-libbers don't see life the same way as Planners. You like to be more flexible—organizing and planning are much too restrictive and rigid. For you, making a list is a waste of time, because you probably won't stick to it anyway. It stifles you. Whereas Planners want organization to make it easier to find things, you have no problem finding something among the scattered mess. In fact, part of the fun is sifting through the stuff, giving you a chance to explore. Besides, you figure that even if it takes you a couple of minutes longer than the Planner to find something, you spent less time putting it away in the first place. That's not to say that you Ad-libbers mind some order, but just not too much of it!

Is anything crystallizing for you yet? If you were to put a check mark next to Planner or Ad-libber for each of the previous categories, which one would have more check marks?

Words that define you. The terms *should* and *ought* seem to guide the actions of you Planners and your expectations of others. They underlie your structured and organized approach to life. They define living by the rules, traditions, and a work ethic. When the work is done, if there's time, you can make some room for play.

You Ad-libbers live more according to such words as "could be," "maybe," and "perhaps." These terms denote flexibility, adaptability, and tolerance—a life that's less structured and more open to opportunity. Your philosophy is to let life happen; you never know when something pleasurable may be around the corner. Even when you work, you'll try to figure out how to make it more fun. Given the choice, you'd rather play before you work and then use a last-minute-rush approach to get the job done.

So after all these descriptions, are you more of a Planner or more of an Ad-libber? Neither one is good or bad. Of course, from the perspective of the Ad-libber, the Planner is too structured, and from the Planner's perspective, the Ad-libber is too spontaneous. Oh well, they say "different strokes for different folks." And that's how you'll decide the right diet plan for you.

Diet Styles

That brings me to the type of eating plan most appropriate for each personality. I want you to read the chapters about each of the plans, even though I'll be making recommendations regarding which plan may be most appropriate for which personality. You may have enough of the characteristics of the opposite personality to find that the eating plan for that personality also works well for you. Also, each eating plan is chock full of great information. The main objective of all of this is for you to find the approach that's most comfortable. I certainly don't want to tell you the eating plan to follow, even though I have found that particular personality types have an easier time with some of the plans than others. I don't know you as you know yourself. Just because it feels right to me doesn't mean it is the right way for you. I think that is the problem with many of the diets on the market today. The author or creator feels really great about the approach and can't seem to figure out why others aren't thinking the same way. We're different and that difference should be honored. My criterion for picking a plan is, if it fits well with who you are, you should be able to follow it for a lifetime and never have a reason to go on a diet again.

This book includes four weight-loss plans:

- The Portion-Control Plan
- The Instead Plan
- The R-U-Hungry Plan
- The Choice Plan

The Portion-Control Plan is a flexible approach that doesn't require much structure. You don't have to keep track of nutrients in the food you eat or do any tallying or keeping of a food diary. Because there are various ways to implement this plan, those of you who like variety might appreciate trying each of them. You can measure your food for a short time so you learn to recognize quantities. You can split everything you eat in half, eating one half and reserving the other half for another meal or to share with someone else. You can also learn to visualize quantities, using everyday objects. We're talking very simple here, which is why you Ad-libbers should be interested.

The Instead Plan is another less structured plan. You get to eat lower-fat, lower-calorie alternatives to your usual foods. A list of substitutes is provided, from which you can select what to eat. This plan should also appeal to the Ad-libber.

The R-U-Hungry Plan may be right for those of you who can "listen to your body talk." This is a plan with little structure, other than asking you to get totally in sync with your body's needs, eating only when you're hungry and stopping as soon as you've reached a satisfied level. Does this sound interesting to you Ad-libbers?

The Choice Plan is a give-me-some-structure-and-I'll-fill-in-the-details approach. It's based on the Boomer's Guide Pyramid. Basically, I'll tell you how many choices you can have from each of the various food groups based on your calorie allowance, and you get to decide what foods you want. For those of you who want more structure, I've even distributed your daily allowances for each meal. Using a simple Choice Tracker, you'll record what you eat. This would be a great approach for you Planners. However, I've had Ad-libbers on this plan for a short time to learn what amounts from each of the food groups is right for them. There's great knowledge here for all types.

Let me reiterate—regardless of whether you're a Planner or an Ad-libber, I want you to select the plan that sounds best to you. You might even try them all. You Ad-libbers should especially like the idea of rotating through all the plans, following each one for about three weeks. The variety will be just what your personality would like.

Because you Ad-libbers enjoy the process more than the completion of a project, changing plans occasionally will keep you energized. I have a theory (and you can tell me if it's right) that, because Ad-libbers enjoy the process so much, whenever they get close to reaching their goal, they subconsciously sabotage their efforts. That may be partly due to thinking that by reaching their goal weight, the process must end. If that's true for you, just remember this—maintaining your new weight is just as much a process as having lost the weight. Maintaining your new healthy lifestyle has to be an ongoing effort.

Another way to make these eating plans interesting is, instead of rotating the plans, try blending them. For example, there's no reason why you can't use the visualizing method of the Portion-Control Plan while you're also doing the Choice Plan. That way you don't have to measure your choices; just visualize what a serving would look like.

What it comes down to is selecting and sticking with whatever works for you.

One last thing to keep in mind: No matter what approach you use, the idea is to establish a healthy relationship with food. It's not the enemy. The main reason for eating is to nourish your body. Keep that in mind when you select foods to eat. It amazes me sometimes how people will take better care of their cars than themselves. If your car requires premium unleaded gas, would you even think to give it regular? Then why isn't the same thought given to what you feed yourself?

I also believe you should enjoy the food you eat. So it comes down to blending the health factor and pleasure factor of eating. First think of what would be healthy foods to eat and then ask yourself, "Which ones would I enjoy from that list?" I'll give you an example. If I offer broccoli, string beans, or zucchini to my oldest daughter, she'll take the first two and reject the last. She just doesn't like zucchini (and believe me, I've tried serving it to her every which way). That's fine, because choosing broccoli or string beans is every bit as healthful for her. My youngest daughter enjoys cauliflower, just not raw cauliflower. I know when I'm serving cauliflower for dinner that I should cook it so she'll eat a healthy vegetable and also enjoy it.

Now you may wonder how this concept of making a healthy list first, then selecting what you'd enjoy can apply to such foods as dessert, treats, chips, and so on. They contain a lot of calories with less nutrition and might not appear on the healthy list. In that regard, I'd say consider what it is you want (let's say, chocolate candy) and think about how much would be healthful for you. Realizing that you're selecting these foods for the pure pleasure of them, their role is not for nourishment. So go easy on them. A bite or two of the chocolate candy bar should satisfy the taste buds without destroying the diet. When you overeat on these foods, you've forgotten the reason to eat—and that is to nourish the body. Tell yourself "I'm eating healthfully. I'm not dieting." Changing the words around like that can do a lot for your mind and attitude.

chapter 15

What Shape Are You in—Apple or Pear?

Middle age is when your age starts to show around your middle.

—Bob Hope

This chapter is not included to make you feel guilty about how much you weigh now. I'm not even concerned how it happened that you're overweight. The past is the past. I want you to look at today as being "the first day of the rest of your life," the beginning of a time when you plan on doing everything in your power to make it a healthy life.

It's time to set some realistic goals. But first, a word of caution to you "pie-in-the-sky" thinkers: Don't go asking for the moon. You want to work toward something that's achievable. If your parents and grandparents were overweight, don't expect to look like the Barbie or Ken doll. On the other hand, don't allow your genetic background to serve as an excuse for not trying to lose weight. There's nothing set in concrete saying you don't have a chance.

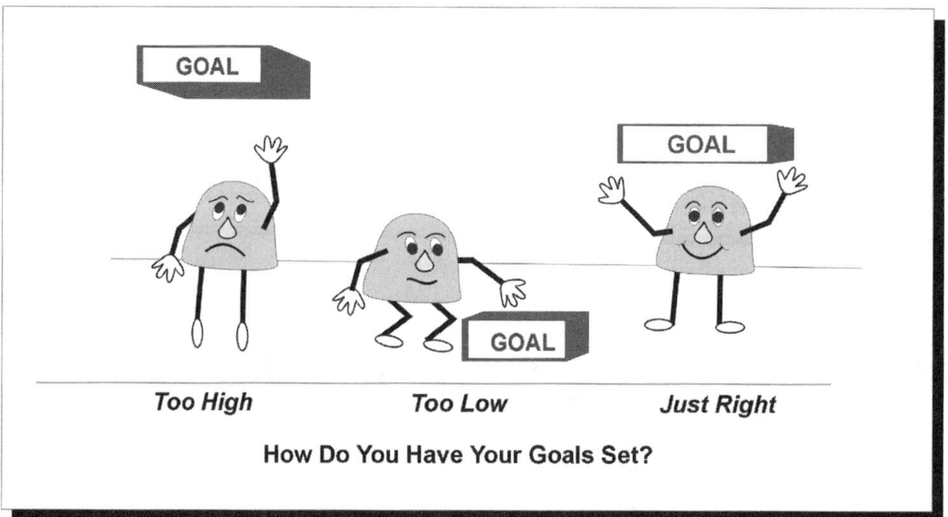

How Do You Have Your Goals Set?

No matter what the weight charts say should be your optimum weight, what you'll end up weighing is going to be based on two things, both of which are totally under your control—how many calories you eat and how much exercise you do. I don't want to hear you say, "But I've got a slow metabolism." To that I reply, "Then rev it up with exercise." Your final weight is going to hinge almost solely on what you're prepared to do and how much commitment you bring to the task. Oh, there will be times that your weight will plateau, where you get stuck at the same weight for what seems like an eternity. So what? Your body is just trying to readjust or find a new setpoint. Is that an excuse to go back to your old habits? No! Ask yourself how committed you are to achieving a lower weight.

The Theory of Setpoint

Whatever your reason for losing weight—whether it's to fit into smaller-size clothes or not be huffing and puffing when you walk up a flight of stairs—your body will seemingly do everything it can to defend its current weight. This is your current setpoint. Your body may be cooperative and allow the first several pounds to come off easily as you start to diet (because most of it will be water loss). However, if you've ever tried to lose weight in the past, you know how difficult it is to get past a certain point.

Your body wants to defend your current weight for a good reason. Programmed into your body's chemistry are ways to protect you during times of famine (and to your body, dieting is like a famine). In the old days, people who could manage with little to no food and hold on to their fat stores were able to survive. Those folks passed on their genetic makeup for this ability to succeeding generations. (So blame your ancestors for some of your weight problem!) When you try to diet, your body responds by slowing down your metabolism, allowing you to manage on less food. That's why you can only go so far with a calorie deficit.

The more fit you are, the easier it is to lose weight. Muscle burns more calories than fat cells do. The more muscle you have, the more calories your body will burn. Because exercise builds muscle, it seems pretty clear to me what you need to do—exercise more. It's a win-win situation. Exercising will burn calories, and your new muscle mass will burn even more calories. It's like compound interest—it builds on itself.

For those of you who aren't the athletic type, your physical activity can be as simple as walking. In fact, brisk walking, a moderate form of exercise done for a prolonged period of time, will burn more calories than an intense workout. Intense exercise uses up the glucose stored in your muscles before going after the fat stored away in your fat cells. Because moderate exercise uses a mix of glucose and fat for energy, you can reduce the size of your fat cells without too much effort. Dieting encourages your body to preserve its fat stores; exercise promotes the reduction of them. I look at nutrition and exercise as though they're a pair of shoes. Would you ever think of going out with only one shoe on? If not, why assume that dieting alone is your answer?

Establishing a new setpoint means you've found the correct balance between how much you eat and how much you need to exercise to maintain the new, lower weight. It will take time because your body has a great memory and, given the chance, it will try to take you back to your old setpoint. However, by the way you eat and exercise, you can show your body who's the boss. Maintaining a new setpoint isn't an overnight event. In fact, you need to maintain your new weight for quite some time in order to be confident that your new weight setpoint is yours to keep.

Setting a Healthy Weight Goal

So how much do you think you should weigh? Is that number based on what would be physically healthy for your body or what the popular size is at the moment? We may have grown up with the likes of Marilyn Monroe and Twiggy setting standards for women, but neither of their figures would make it today. Marilyn Monroe would not be considered fit, and Twiggy would be considered anorexic. At least men had better role models to emulate, such as fitness gurus Jack LaLanne and Arnold Schwarzenegger. The bottom line, though, is that you should determine your weight based on health parameters not on who you want to look like. Enough studies have been done to show at what weight we would increase our risk for disease and at what weight our risk would be low.

Let's do some calculations to find a goal weight for you.

What's your **height** (without shoes)? _______________ inches

What's your **weight** (without clothes)? _______________ pounds

What's the **wrist** measurement of your writing hand? (*Find the bony protrusion or bump on the outside of your wrist. Place a cloth tape measure on your wrist between that bone and your hand. That's the number you want.*) _______________ inches

What's your **waist** measurement? (*Have no clothing around your waist, breathe normally, and stand straight. Place the tape with the measurement scale facing outward. Measure the smallest distance around, below your rib cage and above your belly button. Don't cinch the tape measure or suck in your gut! Make sure that the tape isn't twisted. It's best to measure first thing in the morning.*) _______________ inches

What's your **hip** measurement? (*Measure the widest circumference that includes your butt.*) _______________ inches

Next, you need to determine your **frame size** because it contributes to your overall weight. (I have a small frame and often regret that; it means I can't eat as many calories as someone with a larger frame size who is of the same height.) To find out your frame size, divide your height, in inches, by your wrist measurement, also in inches. The result is your "frame size value."

____________	÷	____________	=	____________
Height (inches)		Wrist Measurement (inches)		Frame Size Value

Now look at the following table. First, locate the column for your gender; then find the frame size value you just calculated. Finally, look to the column at the far right for your frame size. Is that what you thought you were?

Frame Size Value for Females	Frame Size Value for Males	Frame Size
Greater than 11.0	Greater than 10.4	**Small**
10.1 to 11.0	9.6 to 10.4	**Medium**
Less than 10.1	Less than 9.6	**Large**

Source: Your Personality Prescription *by Roberta Schwartz Wennik, M.S., R.D., page 208.*

Frame Sizes

What's your waist-to-hip ratio? Are you pear shaped—carrying a major portion of your weight around your hips—or are you apple shaped—sporting a spare tire around your middle? Even though women complain about their heavy hips, maybe it'll make them feel better to know that fat, when deposited higher up, around the midriff and stomach (which is more typical for men who are overweight), may be an indicator of a higher risk for Type 2 diabetes, hypertension, and cardiovascular disease.

Your hormones have a lot to do with where the fat is deposited. Premenopausal women have high levels of estrogen, which seems to guide extra fat into the hips and thighs. In contrast, because of testosterone, men tend to store away extra fat around their middles. Unfortunately for women, menopause is a time when their estrogen level starts to decline. They may find themselves transforming from pear shaped to apple shaped—that is, unless they alter what they eat and how much physical activity they get. They also are left with less protection against hormone-related diseases. You boomers have time to make the change before most of you hit menopause. Men, even though it's less likely for you to change from apple shaped to pear shaped if you're overweight, you definitely can change your eating and exercise habits.

To determine your waist-to-hip ratio, divide the waist and hip numbers you measured earlier.

____________	÷	____________	=	____________
Waist (inches)		Hips (inches)		Waist-to-Hip Ratio

To be considered apple shaped, a woman would have a waist-to-hip ratio of *greater than or equal to* 0.8, and men would have a ratio of *greater than or equal to* 1.0. Another warning sign of increased risk for a woman is having a waist measurement of greater than 35 inches and for a man to have a 40-inch waist or greater. As you start to lose weight, occasionally take new measurements, realizing that every fraction of an inch decrease and every pound lower are getting you that much closer to lifelong health protection.

The reason I've had you do this bit of calculating is not to keep you busy, but to prepare you for determining your Body Mass Index (BMI). BMI provides you with much more information than your bathroom scale can. Whereas your scale records how many pounds you weigh, the BMI is strongly correlated with total body fat.

Using the following table for BMI, find your height in the leftmost column. Then run your finger across the row to locate your present weight (without clothes). What section of the table did you end up in? Healthy Weight? Overweight? Obese? Keep in mind that the larger a BMI gets past the Healthy Weight range, the greater the health risks, especially if one already has such diseases as heart disease, hypertension, and diabetes.

> People with a Healthy Weight BMI are generally not at risk for any of the major diseases, such as heart disease, diabetes, or cancer. A BMI in the Overweight or Obese range, however, is a red flag saying "lose weight now."

	BODY MASS INDEX[1]													
	19	20	21	22	23	24	25	26	27	28	29	30	35	40
	Weight (in pounds)													
Height	HEALTHY WEIGHT						OVERWEIGHT					OBESE		
4'10"	91	96	100	105	110	115	119	124	129	134	138	143	167	191
4'11"	94	99	104	109	114	119	124	128	133	138	143	148	173	198
5'0"	97	102	107	112	118	123	128	133	138	143	148	153	179	204
5'1"	100	106	111	116	122	127	132	137	143	148	153	158	185	211
5'2"	104	109	115	120	126	131	136	142	147	153	158	164	191	218
5'3"	107	113	118	124	130	135	141	146	152	158	163	169	197	225
5'4"	110	116	122	128	134	140	145	151	157	163	169	174	204	232
5'5"	114	120	126	132	138	144	150	156	162	168	174	180	210	240
5'6"	118	124	130	136	142	148	155	161	167	173	179	186	216	247
5'7"	121	127	134	140	146	153	159	166	172	178	185	191	223	255
5'8"	125	131	138	144	151	158	164	171	177	184	190	197	230	262
5'9"	128	135	142	149	155	162	169	179	182	189	196	203	236	270
5'10"	132	139	146	153	160	167	174	181	188	195	202	207	243	278
5'11"	136	143	150	157	165	172	179	186	193	200	208	215	250	286
6'0"	140	147	154	162	169	177	184	191	199	206	213	221	258	294
6'1"	144	151	159	166	174	182	189	197	204	212	219	227	265	302
6'2"	148	155	163	171	179	186	194	202	210	218	225	233	272	311
6'3"	152	160	168	176	181	102	200	208	216	224	232	240	279	319
6'4"	156	164	172	180	189	197	205	213	221	230	238	246	287	328

Small Frame (BMI 19–21) · Medium Frame (BMI 21–23) · Large Frame (BMI 22–24)

Note: Height is measured without shoes and Weight is measured without clothes.

1. Dietary Guidelines Advisory Committee, 2000 Report and National Institutes of Health, 1998. The BMI (weight-for-height) ranges shown above are for adults. They are not exact ranges of healthy and unhealthy weights. However, they show that health risk increases at higher levels of overweight and obesity. Even within the healthy BMI range, weight gains can carry health risks for adults. Weight-for-frame-size is based on Metropolitan Life Insurance guidelines.

Let's take Sara and Melissa as examples. Sara is 5 foot 6 inches tall and weighs 163 pounds. According to the table, she has an approximate BMI of 26, making her overweight. She needs to lose some weight, especially because she also has high blood pressure. On the other hand, Melissa, who's also 5 foot 6 inches tall, weighs only 138 pounds. With a BMI of 22, she's in the Healthy Weight section. She says she wants to lose weight. Should she?

This is when your *frame size* comes into consideration. Look at the range of weights for each height in the Healthy Weight section. If we continue with the examples of Sara and Melissa, the BMI table says that for their 5'6" height, their weight can range anywhere from 118 pounds to 148 pounds (corresponding to BMIs of 19 to 24). That's a spread of 30 pounds. When the U.S. government created the BMI table, their primary consideration was to classify people according to the health risk their weight posed. A 30-pound range wasn't considered deleterious to one's health. However, I can tell you, depending upon your frame size, those 30 pounds can make a big difference in how you look and feel. I'm 5 foot 4 inches tall, small-framed, and at the low end of the weight range for my height. The table says that I can weigh between 110 and 140 pounds. Only twice in my life have I been about 145 pounds and that was each time I was pregnant with my two daughters. I could not comfortably carry that much weight around normally on my frame size.

It stands to reason that a large-framed person has heavier bones than a person of the same height with a small frame. Those bones obviously contribute to overall weight. Therefore, I thought it would be useful to add another aspect to the BMI table, that of frame size.

Notice that within the Healthy Weight section of the BMI table, a Small Frame includes all the weights with BMIs from 19 to 21. A Medium Frame encompasses all the weights with BMIs from 21 to 23, overlapping some of the weights of the Small Frame. A Large Frame covers weights for BMIs of 22 to 24, again overlapping some of the weights of the Medium Frame. (This is still not an exact science.)

Setting a Goal Is One Thing ... Achieving It Is Another

Sara can see that her 163 pounds or BMI of 26 is too high. With a medium frame, a healthy weight for her can range from 130 to 142 pounds, or a BMI of 21 to 23. Should that be her goal? Yes; but that may be too overwhelming as a long-term goal. She could set some shorter-term goals, first shooting for a BMI of 24, which seems more achievable. That's a loss of just 15 pounds, which should take about 2 to 3 months to accomplish.

When that new setpoint is reached, she can set a new goal of a BMI of 22, and so on.

Do people whose weight occurs in the Healthy Weight section of the BMI table need to lose any weight? Melissa's weight is in the Healthy Weight range. However, when she takes into account her small frame size, her 138 pounds is too heavy. The BMI table says that someone 5 foot 6 inches tall and small framed should be between 118 and 130 pounds. Although there's always a chance for health problems no matter how much you weigh, the risks for major diseases occur at higher rates when people's weight occurs in the Overweight or Obese sections of the table. But losing weight according to your frame size will give you more energy.

> Do you know how to eat an elephant? One bite at a time. Think about that when you set goals that seem too overwhelming. Make them small. They can add up to one big goal in time.

Don't Forget About Body Fat

BMI doesn't tell you your specific percentage body fat. If you want to find that out, you should have a body composition analysis done. When we were younger, a tape measure was all we had to determine how "fat" we were. Now many health clubs offer the service of measuring your body fat, by either hydrostatic weighing (measures weight underwater), bioelectrical impedance (measures resistance of body mass to the flow of a small and harmless electrical current), or skinfold measurement (measures folds of skin and fat with calipers). Because body fat percentage is hard to measure accurately, it's best to take all measurements (waist, hip, frame size, BMI, weight, body fat) into consideration when setting goals and tracking progress.

Most Americans rely on the scale to tell them how they're doing. Yet the scale reflects not only muscle and fat, but also how much water you're retaining. When you're losing weight, how do you know it's the fat you're losing? Body composition analysis can tell you that. There are now home scales that both weigh you and give you your fat percentage. The advantage of monitoring your weight this way is that you can tell if you're losing fat or valuable muscle.

The scale uses bioelectrical impedance analysis. As you stand on the scale barefoot, a low-level electrical current passes through one foot to the other. The scale then measures the resistance, which is a measure of how much fat you have. That's because with fat containing less water than muscle, the current travels more slowly. The scale contains a microchip that takes this information and combines it with your weight and the information you put in about your height and gender. Don't worry that you're going to be fried on the scale. The current is so low that you don't feel it, nor is it harmful. The only people who should be concerned about using it are those who have a pacemaker. If you decide to get one of these scales, read the instructions thoroughly. If you're not completely hydrated or you're overhydrated, the results can be skewed.

Healthy Ranges for Body Fat

	18 to 39 Years	40 to 59 Years	60 to 79 Years
Females	21 to 32%	23 to 33%	24 to 35%
Males	8 to 19%	11 to 21%	13 to 24%

Source: Shape Up America!, 6707 Democracy Boulevard, Suite 306, Bethesda, MD 20817, www.shapeup.org

There's another advantage to knowing your body fat percentage. With it you can be sure that your BMI won't mislead you into thinking you're at an unhealthy weight when you're more muscular—such as is true for bodybuilders and athletes. BMI doesn't distinguish between lean body mass and fat. Although the scale may say you're overweight, you may not be overfat. On the other hand, you could be overfat when the scale says you're at a normal weight. As we age, we tend to get fatter. It doesn't have to be that way. Increasing your physical activity and building your muscle can help slow down the process.

Weighing In

Weighing yourself every day makes no sense. In order to lose 1 pound of body weight, you have to drop 3,500 calories—whether by decreasing your calorie intake, increasing your physical activity, or both (the best option). It must be obvious then that, unless you're eating at least

5,000 calories a day, you can't drop 3,500 calories in food or increase your exercise by that amount in order to lose 1 pound *per day.* (So don't be taken in by those advertisements touting that you can lose 5 pounds in a day!) Besides, it's not even healthful to try. Anything that comes off that quickly goes right back on that quickly. In addition, you would be practically starving yourself and exercising yourself into exhaustion to achieve such an unrealistic goal.

On the other hand, it would be helpful to weigh yourself periodically to see whether you're making any progress. When I say periodically, I mean no more than once a week. Regardless of what the scale says, I can tell you that just the way you look and feel will probably say much more than the scale ever could with much more believability. Even the way your clothes fit will send you similar messages. **If you're eating as healthfully as you can and want to, and you're exercising as much as you can and want to, then you'll end up with the body your efforts produce.** I can't emphasize enough that the level of your success is your choice.

If you do weigh yourself, do so in the morning without any clothes on and after you've gone to the bathroom. It's also best to choose the same day each week on which to weigh yourself. Whatever the scale tells you, don't let the results dictate the way your day is going to go. Don't get emotionally invested in the results. Use those energies to do something constructive to reach your goal.

For those of you who'd like to keep track of your weight-loss progress, Appendix E is a weight-loss log.

chapter 16

How Much Can I Eat?

Never eat more than you can lift.

—Miss Piggy

Now that you have your goal weight determined, it's time to consider how you're going to achieve it. It will require increased physical activity on your part, along with a change in what you eat. You're probably wondering then, how much you'll get to eat. The next several steps will show you an easy way to calculate that.

Step 1: Determine How Many Calories You're Currently Eating

To determine how many calories you're currently eating, you need to assess how active you are. From the following list, decide which level of activity best describes you.

Do most of your work or play activities require you to sit or stand for long periods of time? Do you fit in some physical activity, maybe about once a week? If this sounds like you, your level of activity is sedentary.

Do you tend to be up and about most of the time—doing housework or climbing stairs at work? If you're participating in some form of exercise for at least 30 minutes, 2 to 3 times a week, you can consider your level of activity to be light.

Does your job keep you active? If so, and you're also active in your leisure time for at least 60 minutes, 3 to 5 times a week, you can consider your activity to be at a moderate level.

Does your job involve manual labor? Do you also devote time to aerobic activities during your leisure time for at least five to six times per week? If so, your activity level would probably fall in the active level.

Let me stress how important it is that you assess your exercise level accurately. If you say you're more active than you are, your calorie calculations are going to be too high. You'll be eating too much and you won't be getting much benefit from the weight-loss plan you select.

So how much do you weigh today? Keep that number in mind as I show you how to calculate the approximate number of calories you're presently eating. Look in the left column of the following table to find your usual activity level (based on what you just read). Then look in the appropriate column for your gender, and find the number that will be your "multiplier." Multiply your weight (in pounds) by that number. The result is about how many calories you're eating per day to maintain your present weight.

Multiplier for Calculating Calories

Level of Activity	Women	Men
Sedentary	12	14
Light	13	15
Moderate	14	16
Active	15	17

Let's see what Lori, one of my clients, found out. She rated her activity level as Sedentary. She weighed 160 pounds.

She multiplied her weight by 12, to find out that she was eating about 1,920 calories per day.

David, another one of my clients, admitted to being pretty much a couch potato most of the time. So he rated his activity level as Sedentary. With a weight of 220 pounds, he multiplied that number by 14, to find that his intake was about 3,080 calories per day.

Step 2: Determine Your Calorie Prescription for Losing Weight

There are two ways to come up with a daily calorie level. The first way is called the **80% Rule.** To use this rule, take the number of calories that you just determined you're currently eating and multiply it by 80 percent (or 0.80). The answer you get will be the number of calories you should eat to lose 1 pound per week. Lori discovered that she was eating about 1,920 calories per day. She did the following calculation:

1,920 × 0.80 = 1,536 calories

and found that her daily intake would have to be about 1,500 calories. David did a similar calculation and came up with about 2,500 calories.

Another approach you can use is called the **500-Calorie Rule.** In this case, you subtract 500 calories from the number of calories you're currently eating. When Lori did this calculation, her result was as follows:

1,920 – 500 = 1,420 calories

David's result was 2,580 calories. You could use the lower of the two calorie approaches; that way you err on the conservative side. If you don't want to have to decide which rule to use, you can simply average the results of the two rules.

By reducing your calorie intake by one of the previous amounts, you should lose about 1 pound per week. You may be saying that losing 1 pound per week isn't much. That's because we haven't yet put exercise into the equation. The best body-fat burning is done with moderate activity (something discussed in more detail in Chapter 29). With regular exercise, losing 1½ to 2 pounds per week is quite achievable.

There's one other important rule to remember. If you're a woman, you shouldn't eat fewer than 1,200 calories per day, and if you're a man, you shouldn't eat fewer than 1,500 calories per day. This is true even though your calculations say you should be eating less. At calorie levels that are too low, you run the risk of not getting adequate nutrition. To be on the safe side, I recommend taking a daily multivitamin, with minerals, that has no more than 100 percent Daily Value.

If Your Weight Loss Seems to Plateau

It happens very often that during the process of losing weight, people reach a plateau where they can't seem to lose any more. The whole process seems to come to a screeching halt. You've lost some weight, but your body seems to have reached a state of equilibrium. That's okay; let it! You need to give your body a chance to adjust to this new level and become comfortable with it. To drastically cut calories now would be to put your body into a "stall" mode. You'll slow down your metabolism. The best thing you can do for now is continue with the plan you're on. Closely monitor your weight to be sure you're not putting the lost weight back on. If you start to gain back some weight, remember that 2 or 3 pounds is acceptable, because some of that may be water weight. Continue this way for about several months, and pat yourself on the back if you're able to maintain this level.

After holding that previous level, it's time to get going again. First, weigh yourself to find out what your current weight is. Then, using the appropriate multiplier from the preceding "Multiplier for Calculating Calories" table, recalculate your present calorie intake. (I'm hoping that this time, because you've become more active, you'll be able to use a higher multiplier.) Again using the 80% Rule or the 500-Calorie Rule, calculate what your new calorie intake level should be. It's possible that it could be the same or even higher. If that's the case, I recommend you remain at the same calorie level you're at now and increase your activity—either the intensity of the exercise or the length of time you do it. Let exercise get you over the hump.

Reassess your calorie needs as you see fit. If you haven't yet reached your goal weight, but the new calculations say to eat fewer calories, then eat fewer calories. You'll be edging yourself closer to what will be your maintenance calorie level.

Maintaining Your Goal Weight

Reaching your goal weight is one thing. Being able to maintain that weight is something else. At this point, you want to establish a new setpoint that your body will protect when you occasionally eat too much or exercise too little. The difficulty with having been overweight is that it takes some time to establish a new setpoint. That's why, although reaching your goal weight is commendable, your vigilance can't stop (not yet, and maybe never, depending upon how well your body takes to its new weight). It takes time. At this point, interestingly enough, after you've reached your goal weight, you have your body on your side. What I mean by that is, if you mentally start making up excuses why you can't exercise or eat right, your body will let you know you're slipping. It'll feel lethargic, stiff, and actually cry out for movement. Your energy level will dwindle and your clothes will feel slightly snug. So listen to your "body talk."

chapter 17

The Portion-Control Plan

My doctor told me to stop having intimate dinners for four. Unless there are three other people.

—Orson Welles

It seems America has a preoccupation with *what* we should be eating. There are debates about whether we should be eating high-protein diets or high-carbohydrate diets. Yet what is most important is how *much* we are eating. Portion sizes have gotten out of control, whether we're eating out or eating at home. In fact, studies written up in the January 2003 issues of the *Journal of the American Medical Association* and the *Journal of the American Dietetic Association* showed that portion sizes increased significantly between 1977 and 1996 for many foods. The greatest increase for boomers was for soft drinks, coffee, tea, fruit drinks, beer, ready-to-eat cereals, and foods eaten at fast-food establishments (such as hamburgers and french fries).

Most of us seem to have "stomachs that are bigger than our eyes." Coming from the "clean-your-plate" generation, no matter how much is on our plate it is going to be eaten. So learning to control portion sizes is a definite plus in losing weight. When you think about it, the TV dinners we grew up with provided portion control in compartmentalized trays. In later years, Swanson ruined it by coming out with the Hungry Man Dinner. There went the portion control. Even the so-called "diet" foods have increased their portion sizes. Go to a fast-food restaurant today and they can "supersize" your meal for just pennies more. What a deal! Or is it?

Portion distortion is happening all around us. Bagels are twice as large as they used to be. Muffins now come in such huge muffin cups that at least three people could eat off of. Even the size of the apples in the market are bigger than one serving. (At least I'm less concerned about your eating a little extra fruit.) Eight ounces has always been a standard serving size for beverages. However, a can of soda is 12 ounces and larger. Somehow, people figure that if that's the amount served to them, that's a serving size.

I've eaten at a restaurant that boasts of its mile-high cake. One piece measures about 7 to 8 inches high. You know it has to be a pretty big piece to stay standing all the way from the kitchen to your table. In the 1950s, McDonald's offered only one size of french fries. That size is now their "small." Studies have shown that when people are given larger servings and allowed to eat as much as they want, they eat more. It used to be said that "one's eyes are bigger than one's stomach," meaning you thought you could eat it, but found out you couldn't. People are now proving that saying wrong by showing they can get their stomach to accommodate to the longing of their eyes.

The Portion-Control Plan presented here is great for the person who doesn't want to count calories or grams of fat or look up nutrient values in a list. I have found that this approach is especially suited for the Adlibber, one who doesn't want too much structure in a diet plan. With this method, you don't even have to change your way of eating. However, I hope that you will read the Choice Plan and get some ideas on how to select foods from all the food groups. (Also, don't forget what I shared with you in Chapters 2 and 3 about the pyramid approach to eating.)

The concept behind this plan is quite simple. You have a choice of three ways to do the Portion-Control Plan:

- Measure what you plan to eat.
- Cut everything you plan to eat in half, reserving one half for later or to share with someone.
- Visualize a serving size as your way of apportioning your servings.

See? I didn't say anything about giving up your favorite foods. However, this plan does require some common sense on your part. I want you to appreciate that you can mix and match these methods. You're not stuck with just one. Try one on one day and another the next day. Ad-libbers often enjoy variety, so give all the methods a try.

What's on Your Plate?

The next time you sit down to a meal, take a good look at your plate. What's on it? How much is on it? How crowded are the foods on your plate? Is there any space in between the foods? Many people may be making healthy food choices, but not applying the same philosophy to food portions.

> Too much of a good thing is not a good thing. As Mary Poppins said in the movie of the same name, "A taste is as good as a feast." Keep that in mind as you learn to do the Portion-Control Plan.

The accompanying figure shows a typical American meat-and-potatoes dinner. Not only is the meat taking up at least 50 percent of the plate (probably amounting to a 10 to 12 ounce piece of meat), but the remainder of the plate is filled with starches and fat (mashed potatoes with butter, green peas, and a roll). As you will learn in Chapter 20, peas and potatoes are part of the Starch food group, not the Vegetable group. Therefore, this plate is missing vegetables.

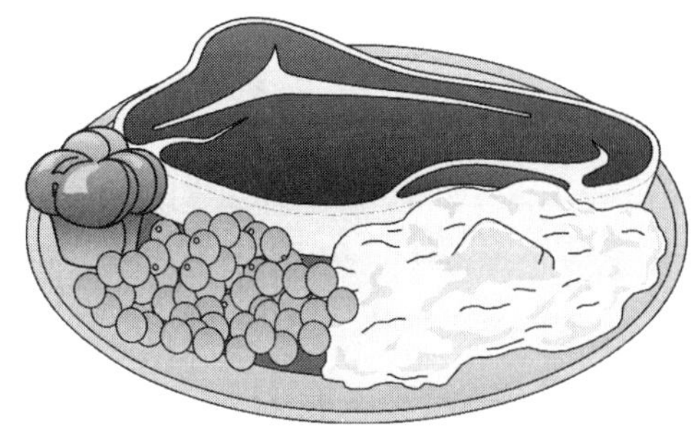

Meat-and-potatoes plate. Does your plate look like this?

The following figures show what I hope your plate will eventually look like.

The meat and fish in these pictures amount to about a 4- to 6-ounce serving. A baked potato or corn on the cob replaces the mashed potatoes (which are often made with cream and fat). Topping the baked potato or corn with a pat of low-fat margarine instead of butter will give you less saturated fat. You could substitute whole-grain brown rice or pasta for the potato or corn. Broccoli or vegetable medley takes the place of the green peas. (If you really wanted the peas, consider them your Starch instead of the potato or corn.) If you prefer, you could have string beans, cabbage, or any other dark green vegetable. The tomatoes provide a nice cold side to the dish and add a little extra color, along with some healthful nutrients.

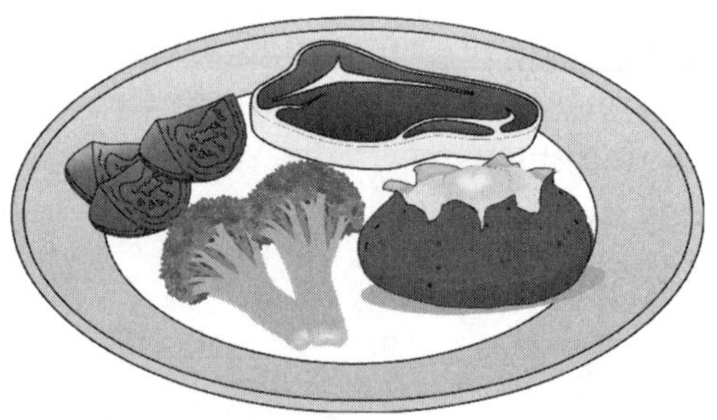

A picture-perfect plate.

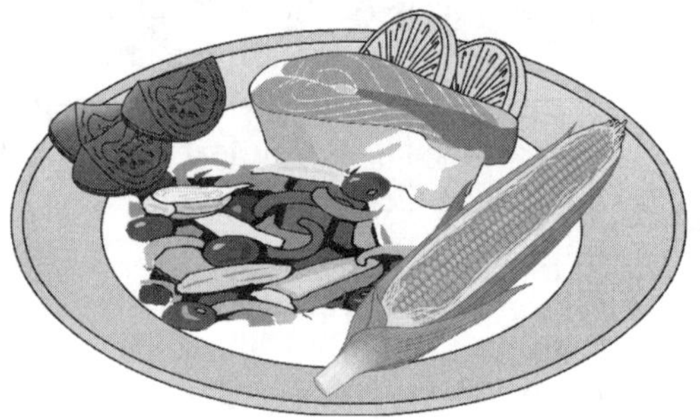

Another picture-perfect plate.

The basic premise behind portion control is making sure you're not eating too much. No matter what method of the Portion-Control Plan you decide is best for you, making healthier choices is still important. For now, though, we'll focus on how to judge what is the right amount to eat.

The Measuring Method

Do you have a kitchen scale and measuring cups? If not, you can purchase them in the kitchen department of a major department store or at a specialty kitchen shop. If you eat out a great deal, this approach may be challenging. You might want to try one of the other two methods instead.

First Week

For the first week, serve yourself the amount you would normally eat. Don't change anything. Be honest! I'm not watching, and this is a learning experience for you. If you have a camera handy, take a picture of your plate. Otherwise, make a sketch by tracing the outline of your plate on a piece of paper. Then draw in the areas occupied by the various foods on your plate. A sketch of the typical American meat-and-potatoes dinner that you saw earlier in this chapter would look like what is shown in the following figure.

Now that you've served yourself with what are your normal portions, measure each food item, using either the scale or measuring cups, as appropriate. There's a form in Appendix E called Portion-Control Log—My Usual Amounts. Use this log to enter your measurements (include units—ounces or cups). See the example in the following table. Again, do this for one week. If you're an Ad-libber, I understand this may seem too structured for you. But what we're after here is for you to get a general idea of what and how much you eat. Let your adventurous spirit have fun with it. This is not a life sentence.

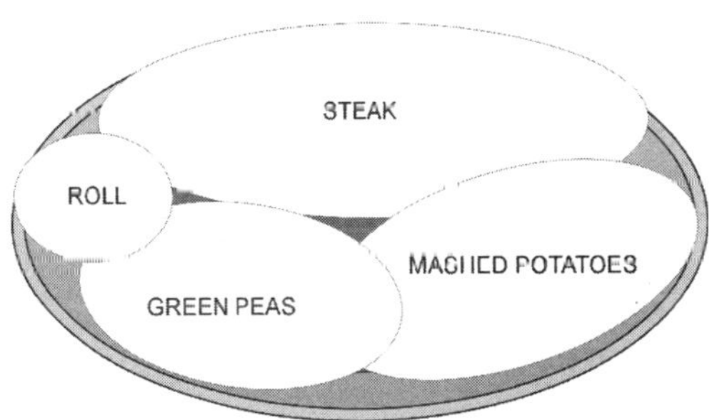

Sketch of the meat-and-potatoes plate.

Jim's Portion-Control Log—Usual Amounts

Date ____________

Meal	Food	Amount (Cups, Ounces)	Standard Serving Size
Breakfast	English muffin	1 muffin	½ muffin
	Butter	3 teaspoons	1 teaspoon
	Orange juice	8 ounces	4 ounces
	Bacon	5 strips	3 strips
	Scrambled eggs	2 eggs	1 egg
	Milk, 1%	1 cup	1 cup
Snack	Pretzels	1½ cups	½ cup

continues

Meal	Food	Amount (Cups, Ounces)	Standard Serving Size
Lunch	Ham and cheese sandwich		
	White bread	2 slices	1 slice
	Cheese	2 ounces	1 ounce
	Ham	4 ounces	2 ounces
	Mayonnaise	3 teaspoons	1 teaspoon
	Apple	1 fruit	1 fruit
	Milk, 1%	8 ounces	8 ounces
Snack	Chocolate chip cookies (4-inch diameter)	2 cookies	1 cookie
	Banana (about 8 inches)	1 fruit	1/2 fruit
Dinner	Steak	10 ounces (cooked)	3 ounces (cooked)
	Mashed potatoes	1 1/2 cups	1/2 cup
	Green peas	1 cup	1/2 cup
	Applesauce	1 cup	1/2 cup

In the example, Jim's log shows what he ate for the day and how much. In the rightmost column, Jim included the standard serving size for each of the foods he ate. When it comes time for you to record what you eat, the following table will give you an idea of what is considered a serving based on food-labeling standards.

Standard Serving Sizes for the Boomer's Guide Pyramid

Food Group	What Counts as a Serving?
Bread, cereal, rice, and pasta	1 slice bread
	1/2 bagel, hamburger bun, or English muffin
	1 small roll, biscuit, or muffin
	5 to 6 small crackers
	3/4 cup ready-to-eat cereal

Food Group	What Counts as a Serving?
	3/4 cup cooked cereal, rice, or pasta
	1 small potato
Vegetable	1 cup raw leafy vegetables
	1/2 cup other vegetables, cooked or chopped raw
	1/2 cup vegetable juice
Fruit	1 medium apple, banana, orange
	1/2 cup chopped, cooked, or canned fruit (in light syrup or natural juice)
	1/2 cup fruit juice
	1/4 cup dried fruit
Dry beans and legumes	1/2 cup cooked beans, peas, or legumes
Milk and yogurt	1 cup milk
	8 ounces of yogurt
Meat, poultry, eggs, and cheese	Meat and poultry: 3 to 4 ounces
	Eggs: 1
	Nuts: 1 ounce (approximately 6 to 10 nuts)
	Nut butter: 2 tablespoons
	Cheese: 1 ounce
	Cottage cheese: 1/4 cup
Fish	3 to 4 ounces
Fats	Butter, margarine, oil, mayonnaise: 1 teaspoon
	Salad dressing: 1 tablespoon
Sweets	Varies according to the sweet. Check out Appendix H.

Note: A few serving sizes have been adjusted to agree with those suggested in the Choice Plan.

After you've done your log for a week, circle the foods that were greater than a standard serving size. As you can see from Jim's example, he went way over. That's okay. This is just the learning stage for now.

There's a difference between "portion size" and "standard serving size." The Food Guide Pyramid, as well as food labels, provides standard serving sizes determined and set by the USDA. Portion size is based on what you choose to eat. For example, when you have a plate of spaghetti, you might say you're having "one serving"; based on the standard serving size of 3/4 cup, however, your portion of 3 cups is more like 4 servings.

Second Week

For your second week, I want you to measure your food for all your meals according to the standard serving sizes. If a standard serving for a food is 1/2 cup, then 1/2 cup of that food is all you get. Pay close attention to how the food fits and looks on the plate. Use your regular dishes—you'll need to get a good idea of how standard serving sizes appear on them. Again, use the Portion-Control Log, jotting down what you ate and how much you served yourself. For one of your meals, take a picture or sketch the areas the food takes up on your plate.

Third Week

During the third week, you'll be working on making healthier choices. Although portion size is what we're working on here, the food choices you make are every bit as important. Look over your logs. Are all the food groups represented? (Chapters 3 and 20 will help you here.) The Choice Plan that is covered soon will give you an idea of how many servings you should have from each food group, based on your calorie needs. After you've read that chapter, review your logs to see whether you're getting enough or too much.

What do you think about the Measuring Method? Does it sound like something you would be willing to do? This isn't something that you'll have to do forever. After you've gotten a feel for what quantities look like, you won't have to measure everything all the time. Of course, it wouldn't hurt to revisit the method occasionally to be sure your portions aren't slowly getting larger.

The Splitting Method

Another approach to the Portion-Control Plan is to divide your serving into two equal halves, putting half away for another day or sharing it with someone. I want to show you what a difference this one little step can make. Serve yourself your usual portion. Now divide each food item on your plate in half. Measure how much you have remaining on your plate. (You'll only have to do this once to see how effective this simple method can be.) Look in Appendix E for the Portion-Control Log—One Half My Usual Amount Log. Write down your results. Again, include the standard serving sizes for the foods you eat. How do the two compare? In our example, look at Jim's log that follows. You can see how much closer he came to the standard serving size with this simple exercise. (By the way, because a whole apple and 8 ounces of milk are standard serving sizes, he didn't have to halve those amounts.)

Jim's Portion-Control Log—One Half Usual Amount

Date ________________

Meal	Food	Original Amount (Ounces, Cups)	One Half Original Amount	Standard Serving Size
Breakfast	English muffin	1 muffin	1/2 muffin	1/2 muffin
	Butter	3 teaspoons	1 1/2 teaspoons	1 teaspoon
	Orange juice	8 ounces	4 ounces	4 ounces
	Bacon	5 strips	2 1/2 strips	3 strips
	Scrambled eggs	2 eggs	1 egg	1 egg
	Milk, 1%	1 cup	1 cup	1 cup
Snack	Pretzels	1 1/2 cups	3/4 cup	1/2 cup
Lunch	Ham and cheese sandwich			
	White bread	2 slices	1 slice	1 slice
	Cheese	2 ounces	1 ounce	1 ounce
	Ham	4 ounces	2 ounces	2 ounces

continues

Meal	Food	Original Amount (Ounces, Cups)	One Half Original Amount	Standard Serving Size
	Mayonnaise	3 teaspoons	1½ teaspoons	1 teaspoon
	Apple	1 fruit	1 fruit	1 fruit
	Milk, 1%	8 ounces	8 ounces	8 ounces
Snack	Chocolate chip cookie (4-inch diameter)	2 cookies	1 cookie	1 cookie
	Banana (about 8 inches)	1 fruit	½ fruit (about 4.5-inch banana)	½ fruit (about 5-inch banana)
Dinner	Steak (cooked)	10 ounces	5 ounces	3 ounces
	Mashed potatoes	1½ cups	¾ cup	½ cup
	Green peas	1 cup	½ cup	½ cup
	Applesauce	1 cup	½ cup	½ cup

Even though you won't be keeping track of calories, I want to point out the value of this one easy step of cutting everything you eat in half. The original amount of food Jim served himself for the day in the log contained 4,000 calories. Halving the portion sizes he served himself gave him a saving of 2,000 calories. This also brought him closer to standard serving sizes. Best of all, it was done with little effort.

Do I hear some of you saying, "I'll feel deprived because I'm not getting to eat both halves? The other half is sitting there in the refrigerator calling out to me." You may find cutting everything in half too drastic a change for you, because you feel hungry all the time. (Be sure that the hunger isn't in your mind rather than your stomach.) Then start by removing only one third of the amount you normally eat, instead of cutting everything in half. Obviously, you'll lose weight more slowly. However, I'd rather you lose weight comfortably than abandon the approach because your hunger is not being satisfied. After continuing with this amount for a couple of weeks, try removing some more—moving up to half your usual amount. What you're trying to do is make a smooth transition to the optimum portion amount.

As with the Measuring Method, take a picture of or sketch what your plate looks like before you make any changes. Then, once you've split it (whether it be by one half or one third), take another picture or draw another sketch. As you serve yourself, your portions should approximate your "new" picture. Occasionally look at your sketch and see how you're doing. Have your amounts crept back to their original size? Time to start splitting again.

Dining Out

When you dine out, you can easily apply portion control. In fact, if you don't, you'll end up overeating. Restaurants rarely serve standard serving sizes. Most patrons would be angry paying high restaurant prices for a 4-ounce serving of meat. (On the other hand, if you're eating in an elegant five-star restaurant, it's considered *haute cuisine* to be served less food on a larger plate. And you get to pay many dollars for the privilege!) The best way to approach these large servings is to have your server bring you a doggie bag at the time your meal is served, not at the end. Practice your portion control—cut your meal in half and put one half in the doggie bag before you've tasted anything. You've saved yourself many calories, and now you get to have a second dinner from that restaurant meal tomorrow night for the same price. (Just think, you've even saved yourself having to cook the next night.)

If you can't imagine having to give up anything as you have to do with the Splitting Method, then the Measuring Method (as discussed earlier) or the Visualizing Method (coming up next) may be better. With these other methods, you serve yourself the correct amount to begin with.

The Visualizing Method

There will be times when you either aren't in the position to measure your food (for example, when you're dining out) or you simply don't want to. That's when the Visualizing Method comes in handy. Using some visual models of everyday objects, you can approximate a standard serving size of the food.

For example, when cutting off a serving from a brick of cheese, try to imagine four dice lined up. That should be equivalent to about 1 ounce cheese. If you have some dice, try it. Now weigh the amount of cheese you've cut. How close did you come to 1 ounce? If you want some margarine on your toast, use the tip of your thumb to approximate 1 teaspoon. Making pancakes for breakfast? Compare the size you make with a compact disc (CD). Are yours too big, too small, or just right? I'm sure you get the idea.

Use the following pictures to help you with the Visualizing Method.

Everyday Objects for Food Portion Comparisons

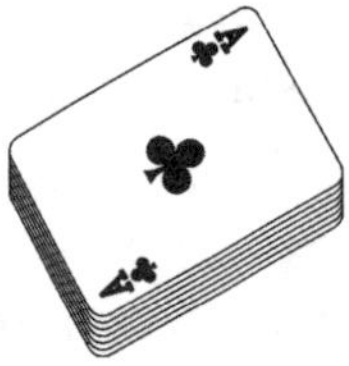

Deck of cards = 3 ounces of cooked meat

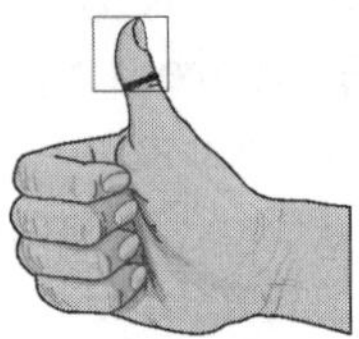

Tip of your thumb = 1 teaspoon

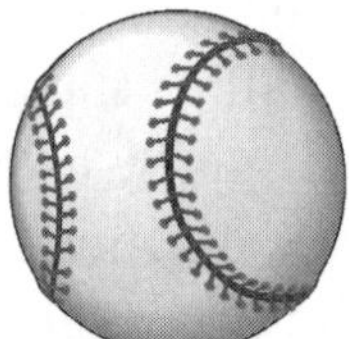

Baseball = 1 cup

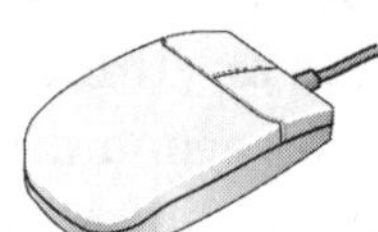

Computer mouse = 1 potato

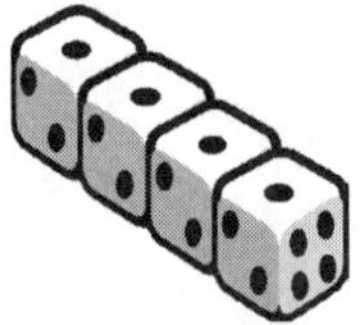

4 dice = 1 ounce of cheese

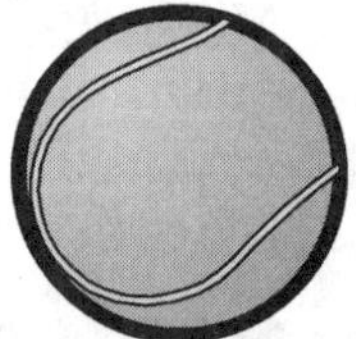

Tennis ball = 1/2 cup or 1 medium apple or peach

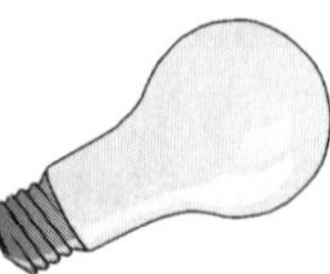

Light bulb = 1 serving of broccoli

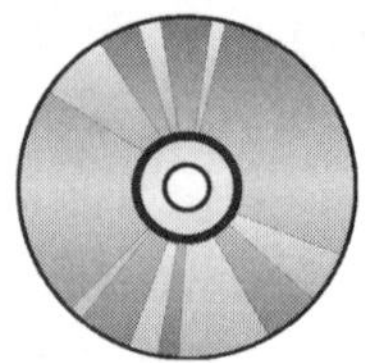

Compact disc (CD) = 1 pancake

Reading food labels becomes very important with this approach. As you look at the label, see whether you can visualize the serving sizes stated in the Nutrition Facts. After you've served yourself using everyday objects as models, measure them with measuring cups and spoons. Did the amount you served yourself agree with what was on the label? Do this little exercise for about a week while you learn to recognize quantities. After that, all you need to do is visualize the object when either you serve yourself the food or have to decide how much to eat when you dine out.

At first glance, you may not be sure whether any of these methods is right for you. I suggest you try them and see. You may be pleasantly surprised. Of course, if the Portion-Control Plan isn't for you, there are a number of other methods in this book that should work.

chapter 18

The Instead Plan

I can resist everything except temptation.
—Oscar Wilde

Many of our food choices are based on habit or tradition. For breakfast, do you think your eggs are too lonely on the plate without bacon? For a snack, do you partake in the doughnuts or other sweets someone always brings into work? Is lunch invariably fast food? Would you think of having a hamburger without french fries? Is a bedtime snack part of your nightly ritual? The choices you've been making are done without much forethought. They're habits.

Now that you've decided to lose weight, the question is how? If you're like many others, the thought of having to totally overhaul your way of eating, eliminating everything that you like, sounds too objectionable to even consider trying. However, if I told you that all you had to do was choose healthier substitutes for some of your favorite high-calorie, high-fat, high-sugar, low-fiber foods, would you be interested? You won't even have to count calories or grams of fat.

This is another plan that should appeal to the Ad-libber who wants both very little structure and the freedom to decide what to eat and how much. With that freedom comes a big responsibility, though. The number of pounds you lose will be very much based on how often you select the healthier alternatives to your favorite foods. It works well, whether you're doing the cooking or eating out. (See Chapters 27 and 28 for more ideas on dining out.)

By the way, Planners, don't think I've forgotten you. Even though I may mention that a particular plan may work for an Ad-libber, that isn't to say that it wouldn't work for you. That's why I want everyone to read all of the plans and choose what sounds agreeable to them.

Although I provide lists of alternative foods, it does help to consider how you put your meals together. The Choice Plan coming up should serve as a healthy format for the Instead Plan. Read it so you have some idea how many servings of each food group you should have for your daily calorie allowance.

How It Works

Let's say that your usual breakfast includes a banana, a doughnut, a cheese omelet, and whole milk. Your choices are high in fat and low in fiber. With some minor changes and alternative selections, your breakfast could be similar but healthier. The banana is a good choice, so leave it in. *Instead* of the doughnut, have a low-fat bran muffin. *Instead* of the cheese omelet, have a scrambled egg made with a vegetable oil cooking spray, and sprinkle on a little cheese-flavored butter substitute flakes. *Instead* of whole milk, have 1 percent or skim milk. Your basic breakfast plan is the same; only the calories, fat, and fiber have changed—for the better.

Of course, there may be times when alternatives are not available. In those cases, consider selecting something entirely different, or eat less of the available food. In other words, use portion control.

Great Choices

The lists that follow are only suggestions. It doesn't mean that when you eat your usual choices, you're being bad or your weight-loss plans are doomed. Just realize that the more times you eat the alternatives, the faster you'll reach your goal weight. If you're on a restricted-sodium diet, then look for reduced-sodium versions of foods.

Instead of This ...	Try This
	Starches
Baked potato with all the trimmings	Small baked potato with low-fat or nonfat sour cream, chives, sprinkle of bacon-flavored butter substitute flakes
	Small baked potato topped with salsa
Buttered popcorn	Air-popped popcorn sprayed with butter-flavored vegetable oil cooking spray; sprinkled with flavored butter substitute flakes
	Ready-to-eat cereal
Buttered toast	Toast spread with a small amount of jam, jelly, or apple butter
	Toast drizzled with olive oil and balsamic vinegar
Croissant	Mexican or Hawaiian sweet bread
Cinnamon bun	Soft pretzel, sprayed with butter-flavored vegetable oil cooking spray and sprinkled with cinnamon and sugar (or sugar substitute)
French fries	Baked potato chips
	Crisp pickle chips
	Baked julienne cut potatoes sprayed with vegetable oil cooking spray and seasoned to taste
Pancakes or waffles with butter and syrup	Pancakes or waffles topped with low-fat yogurt and fresh fruit
Pasta	Whole-wheat pasta
Potato chips	Baked potato chips
	Pretzels
	Baked bagel, tortilla, or pita chips
	Low-fat crackers
	Nonbuttered popcorn
	Crisp pickle chips
	Ready-to-eat cereal

Instead of This …	Try This
Snack crackers (often high in fat)	Melba toast
	Low-fat crackers
	Rice cakes
	Matzo
	Bread sticks
Sugared ready-to-eat cereals	Ready-to-eat nonsugared cereals with at least $2\frac{1}{2}$ grams fiber per serving; add sugar substitute if you want a sweet taste
	Hot oatmeal (If on a salt-restricted diet, avoid instant cereal.)
	Check label for serving size, which can vary greatly between cereals.
White bread	Whole-grain breads (preferably with at least $1\frac{1}{2}$ grams fiber).
	Whole grain should be the first ingredient listed. Limit fat to 2 grams per serving.
White rice	Brown rice.
	Bulgur.
	You can cut your sodium intake by cooking grains without salt.
	Vegetables
Avoiding fresh vegetables because you think they're too much work to clean and cut up	Cut-up vegetables (carrots, celery, broccoli, cauliflower) available in the produce department of your market
	Frozen vegetable medley
Canned vegetables	If you need to restrict your sodium intake, drain and rinse the vegetables before heating.
	Look for "no salt added" varieties.
	Frozen vegetables, which taste closer to fresh than canned vegetables do
Creamed corn	Corn on the cob (If you want, use spray margarine.)
Frozen vegetables in butter sauce	Plain frozen vegetables—add salsa, fresh herbs, or a sprinkle of lemon juice and grated Parmesan cheese

Instead of This …	**Try This**
Iceberg lettuce	Romaine lettuce Green leafy lettuce Cabbage Organic greens Spinach
Mashed potatoes made with cream and butter	Make your mashed potatoes with skim milk or nonfat half-and-half. Sprinkle with butter-flavored or bacon-flavored butter substitute flakes. Top your potato with low-fat cottage cheese.
	Fruits
Sweetened applesauce	Unsweetened applesauce with sugar substitute
Canned fruit in heavy syrup	Canned fruit in natural juices or water Eat just the fruit and discard the heavy syrup. Fresh fruit
Fruit juice	Whole fruit—you get more fiber and fewer calories. One orange is the same as 4 ounces of juice, which may not be as satisfying.
Fruit nectar	Fruit juice (fewer calories and less sugar)
Fruit drinks	Fruit juice (fewer calories and less sugar)
	Dairy
Cheeses	Low-fat varieties (fewer than 5 grams of fat per ounce) Fat-free varieties Strong cheeses such as gorgonzola, goat, and blue deliver more flavor; therefore, you need less.
Mozzarella, whole milk	Mozzarella, part skim milk
Ricotta cheese, whole milk	Ricotta cheese, part skim milk
Cottage cheese, 2% fat	Cottage cheese, 1% fat or nonfat
Cream (for whipping)	Nondairy whipped topping
Cream cheese	Neufchatel Low-fat cream cheese Fat-free cream cheese

Instead of This ...	Try This
Half-and-half	Fat-free half-and-half Evaporated skim milk Nondairy creamers (regular or flavored)
Sour cream	Lite sour cream Fat-free sour cream Low-fat or nonfat yogurt
Whipped cream	Whipped evaporated skim milk Low-fat frozen nondairy whipped topping
Whole milk	Wean yourself from whole milk by first trying 2% reduced milk, moving on to 1% low-fat milk, and then finally switching to skim milk. Soy milk.
	Meats and Eggs
Beef (highest to lowest fat content—"Choice" grade): Regular ground beef, brisket, untrimmed and highly marbled cuts, ribs, sirloin, rib eye steak, London broil, blade roast, porterhouse steak, T-bone steak	Beef (lowest to highest fat content—"Select" grade): Eye of round, top round, tip roast, bottom round, top loin steak, arm roast, tenderloin, flank Try to choose hamburger that is extra lean (about 9% on the label). The leanest cuts of beef are the parts that get the most exercise ("chuck" from the neck and shoulder, "shank" from the lower leg, "flank" from the belly, "round" from the upper back leg. These cuts have more muscle and less fat, which means you need to cook them longer to tenderize them. Use moist-heat methods, such as braising and stewing.) Select meat with less marbling. Cook with fat left on edge to maintain moisture, but remove before eating. Trim away as much as possible. Marinate lower-fat cuts of meat in juice, wine-flavored vinegar, or fat-free dressings to tenderize and optimize juiciness. For tender cuts from the loin, try such low-fat cooking methods as broiling, grilling, or roasting on a rack.

Instead of This ...	Try This
	Veal: top round, leg cutlet, arm steak, sirloin steak
	Moose, elk, bison, antelope, deer, wild rabbit
Cheese omelet	Scrambled eggs made with vegetable oil cooking spray and seasoned with herbs and flavored butter substitute flakes Omelet stuffed with veggies Try salsa on your eggs Poached egg
Chicken or turkey: leg, thigh, cuts with skin	Breast, cuts without skin. Remove skin before eating. Leaving skin on while cooking will keep it moister.
Frankfurters—beef and/or pork	Frankfurters—turkey or chicken (Check label to be sure lower in fat.)
Fried fish	Poached or grilled fish Salmon, tuna, mackerel, sea trout, bluefish, herring, and anchovies are especially rich in the heart-protective omega-3 fatty acids.
Hamburger, ground beef	Ground turkey breast
Lamb: Untrimmed cuts, rib chop, sirloin roast	Lamb: shank leg, shoulder roast, trimmed cuts, loin chop, blade chop
Meat	4 ounces tofu cut up into stir-fry 4 ounces grilled firm tofu ½ cup cooked dry beans (kidney, pinto, navy), split peas, or lentils. (Canned beans help save time.)
Pork: Untrimmed cuts, spareribs, shoulder blade steak, loin rib chop, sirloin roast, sausage, bacon	Pork: tenderloin, top loin roast, top loin chop, back loin ribs, Canadian bacon, ham
Pressed sandwich meats, such as bologna or picnic loaf	Lean sandwich meats: ham, turkey (preferably breast), or beef
Prime grade (normally only available in restaurants)	Select or Choice grades (Select is lowest in fat)
Sausage	Vegetarian-style sausage or turkey sausage (baked or prepared with vegetable oil cooking spray)

Instead of This ...	Try This
Tuna canned in oil	Tuna canned in water
Whole egg	2 egg whites Egg substitute
	Fats and Sauces
Butter	Margarine (with liquid vegetable oil listed first in ingredients) Butter-flavored vegetable oil cooking spray Butter-flavored butter substitute flakes Peanut butter Canola oil, olive oil, safflower oil Jelly
Coconut milk	1% low-fat milk flavored with coconut extract
Cream soup	Minestrone or vegetable soup Broth Soup prepared with nonfat half-and-half
Gravy	Defatted au jus (Chill meat drippings and then remove layer of fat.)
Margarine, stick	Margarine, tub (less saturated and trans fats) Margarine without trans fats
Mayonnaise	Reduced calorie or nonfat mayonnaise Mustard
Oil for frying	Vegetable oil cooking spray and nonstick pan
Roux-based sauce (made with butter and flour)	Try thickening your sauce or gravy with cream of rice cereal. Just a teaspoon or two should do.
Salad dressing	Reduced-calorie or nonfat dressing Favorite dressing or olive oil plus vinegar in a 1:2 ratio Try balsamic vinegar or herbal vinegar for a richer flavor. Lemon juice
Shortening for baking	Replace two thirds of amount required in recipe with applesauce or prune purée.
Tartar sauce	Cocktail sauce

Instead of This ...	Try This
	Treats
Cake, cupcakes, brownies	Angel food cake
Chocolate candy	1 teaspoon fat-free chocolate syrup licked slowly from the spoon Chocolate fudge Jelly beans Miniature marshmallows
Cookies	Animal cookies Fig bars Gingersnaps Graham crackers Vanilla wafers
Normal serving size of cookies is 3 cookies.	Have just 1 cookie or even half a cookie. (You get the flavor and fewer calories. Besides, calories fall out of broken cookies!)
Crumb crust on bakery goods	Top with Grapenuts or fat-free granola cereal.
Doughnuts	Fat-free or low-fat muffins (Watch the size, though, and realize they may be fat free but not sugar free or calorie free.) Whole-wheat toast with jam
Fruit pie	Eat the fruit and leave the crust.
Hard candy	Dried fruit
Ice cream *or* Ice cream sundae	Frozen yogurt Sorbet Sherbet (less fat than ice cream but more sugar) Low-fat ice cream Juice bars
½ cup serving of ice cream	1 tablespoon of ice cream (Think of ice cream as a mouth refresher where 1 tablespoon should be sufficient rather than making the ice cream a meal.)
	Alcohol
Beer, regular	Beer, light
Bloody Mary	Virgin Mary (nonalcoholic Bloody Mary)

Instead of This …	Try This
Eggnog	Mulled cider
Hard-liquor drinks	Wine spritzer (half wine and half club soda or diet soda)
Wine	Sparkling nonalcoholic cider
Soft drinks	Flavored sparkling water Dilute fruit juice with seltzer Add a slice of fresh orange or lime to seltzer or water
	Cooking Methods
Fried	Baked, broiled, grilled, poached, or microwaved
Sautéed in butter	Baked, broiled, or grilled without butter Sautéed in nonstick pan with vegetable oil cooking spray, if necessary Sautéed with a small amount of water or broth Stir-fried
With dressing, sauce, or gravy	Have dressing, sauce, or gravy on the side, and then dip the fork into the dressing first before putting the food on the fork. Add garlic, hot and sweet peppers, fresh ginger, and/or fresh herbs instead of dressing, sauce, or gravy to spice up flavors.

The Instead Plan for Emotional Eating

Another version of the Instead Plan deals with emotional eating—eating when you're bored, stressed, tired, or lonely—but you're not actually hungry. Make up an "Instead" list—things you can do that are not based on food. For example, you might call a friend, write some letters, read a book, work out at the gym, listen to music, take a walk or walk your dog, surf the Internet, or take a bubble bath. When you find yourself reaching for food and you know you're not hungry, consult your list to help you bypass the calories you don't need.

chapter 19

The R-U-Hungry Plan

If hunger makes you irritable, better eat and be pleasant.

—Sefer Hasidim

Stop gritting your teeth to get through the hunger pangs. And stop chewing when there are no hunger pangs. In other words, eat when you're hungry and stop eating when you're not. It's just that simple. The R-U-Hungry Plan is especially suited for those people who are attuned to their inner bodily sensations. The way you would react to the following scenario may tell you a lot about yourself and whether this is the right plan for you.

You've just had a complete breakfast and aren't the least bit hungry. As you pass a bakery, the delicious smells of fresh pastries waft out the door, and in the window you see heaps of jelly-filled doughnuts and chocolate éclairs. Do you pass right on by or are you drawn into the bakery?

If you enter the bakery, you are not listening to your body talk. It didn't give you any signs of being hungry. You're being guided by the pleasure principle (sights and smells), not the hunger principle. To some extent, Americans have been indoctrinated in "opportunistic eating." Everywhere we go, there are food cues. If it's not a fast-food restaurant on every corner, there's an espresso stand (especially if you live in Seattle). On the other hand, if you're willing to walk right on by because you're not hungry, this plan may work for you. Read on and see.

Ad-libbers, if willing to be guided by their hunger, should find this approach easy to follow because there is very little structure. All it takes is a willingness to take the time to recognize whether you're actually hungry. Planners, you, too, will find this plan very effective even if you decide to go with the more structured Choice Plan. There's value to everyone to respond to the needs of their body.

Young children are a perfect example of eating to one's hunger level. Many studies have shown that when children are given access to as much food as they want, they'll stop eating when they're just satisfied. Yet we baby boomers know what it was like growing up with parents who insisted that we clean our plates. Who got a chance to recognize fullness? You just ate until you "made all gone." There's no question that our upbringing has influenced our eating habits. We've lost touch with our body's reaction to what we put in it. You know that's the case when you see all those antacid commercials on television. Why do people insist on eating greasy, spicy foods that cause them such discomfort and then resort to popping antacids to take care of the damage? We're just not listening when our body speaks.

Why People Eat When They're Not Hungry

The reasons people eat when they're not hungry are so numerous that they would probably fill an entire book. Here are some of the more obvious reasons for why we start eating when not hungry or continue eating when we're full:

- A food's smell.
- The sight of food.
- Feeling you always have to have dessert even if you're full just so you can have a sweet taste left in your mouth.
- Being bored.

- Eating to stay awake.
- There's still food left on the plate.
- Trying to satisfy thirst with food.
- Using food as a transition activity—a way of avoiding starting something.
- Using food to deal with emotional issues.
- Fear of not getting a particular food again.
- Food is part of a social activity.
- Eating at a buffet implies you can have at least one of each food.
- Using food as a reward for doing a good job.
- Eating a particular food whenever a specific event occurs (for example, popcorn at the movies).
- Dining with a group of people and they're still eating.
- Feeling you paid for the food, you're going to get your money's worth.
- Wanting to be sure you won't get hungry later when food won't be readily available.
- A friend made you a particular food and you don't want to hurt that person's feelings by not eating it.
- Needing to have that "stuffed" feeling to know the meal is over.
- Serving yourself more than you need to be sure you get enough (for example, serving "family style" or going out for Asian food).
- Not wanting to waste food.
- Not wanting to have leftovers.
- Eating so quickly that your body doesn't recognize how much food it has had.
- With various distractions (conversation, television, and so on), lack of awareness of how much is being eaten.
- Enjoying the flavors so much.
- The food came in a "serving-sized" package.
- Tasting food while you're cooking it.
- Finding that the container you're storing the leftovers in isn't quite large enough, so you eat what doesn't fit.

- You're programmed to eat by the clock.
- Having so much variety of food selections on the plate.
- Eating all foods on a prescribed weight-loss plan because you believe you have to.

Can you add some of your own reasons for starting to eat when you're not really hungry or why you continue eating past being satisfied?

Hunger and Fullness Are Physiological

Do you know how to recognize when you're hungry? For some, it's an obvious stomach growling or grumbling. For others, it might be a slight light-headed feeling, a lack of energy, or an empty feeling. If you're getting dizzy and faint, your blood sugar is probably low and you've waited too long to satisfy that hunger.

Learning to recognize the correct signals can be challenging when trying to overcome other forces. Maybe you're used to eating by the clock (8 A.M.—breakfast; noon—lunch; 6 P.M.—dinner). Or maybe your body has sent you signals, but because you're involved in a project that can't be interrupted, you ignore them. Eventually it seems that the hunger has passed. That's because your liver is doing what it can to deliver glucose into your bloodstream. Just because the hunger signals have passed for a while doesn't mean your body isn't in need of food to replenish the glycogen stores in your liver. The idea behind any weight-loss plan is to nourish your body, not starve it. Some people don't ever experience the sensation of hunger. If that's true for you, this plan may not be the right one.

Do you know when you're full? After you've eaten a little bit of food, your stomach starts to stretch, which sends signals to your brain announcing that food is on its way. It takes about 20 minutes for the food to pass from your mouth through your stomach and on to your intestines. Once there, a hormone called *cholecystokinin* (*koly-sisto-ki-nin*) sends more messages to your brain letting it know that food is now in the intestine and soon can be absorbed. This hormone helps slow

> At your next meal, put your fork down within 20 minutes of starting to eat. Sit still and become aware of your fullness level. Are you just satisfied or are you starting to get too full at this point?

down the emptying of your stomach, causing it to stretch even more and reinforce the messages to your brain. That's why it's so important to *eat slowly*—to allow this process to work efficiently and effectively. Many people eat so fast that they never let the message get to their brain. So they end up overeating.

Have you had the opportunity to visit a warehouse store, such as Costco or Sam's Club, or your supermarket when they're giving out samples? Even though I don't normally recommend you go shopping when you're hungry, try it this once. Go around lunchtime. (That's when there are plenty of samples to try.) Now time how long it takes you from eating your first sample to the last. Because these samples are normally scattered throughout the store, you often have some time between tastes. Many people I've talked with say the same thing: "By the time I left the store, those several samples were enough to fill me up." This is amazing, because the quantity of those samples is far less than what people would normally serve themselves if they were sitting down to eat. What it shows, though, is that when you eat slowly, a small quantity goes a long way to filling you up. That's because you gave your body enough time to let the food register its presence to the brain and then allow the brain to send out its own satiety signals.

Another thing that you should consider is the effect of the food on your taste buds. The first bite of a food is normally the most tantalizing (that is, if you like the flavor of the food). Up until you started eating, your taste buds were, sort to speak, in neutral or asleep. By eating, you have awakened them. However, after repeatedly experiencing the same flavors, the taste buds become satiated or desensitized to the taste. The more slowly you eat, the sooner the taste buds will reach this state. That's why you should ask yourself whether you're still really getting the same pleasure out of the fifth or eighth bite as you did the first.

Gauging Your Hunger and Fullness

Recognizing fullness is just as crucial as being aware of when you're hungry. It's probably even more so, because ignoring fullness signals leads to eating excess calories. The next time you eat, refer to the following hunger-fullness gauge to find out where your hunger needle is pointing.

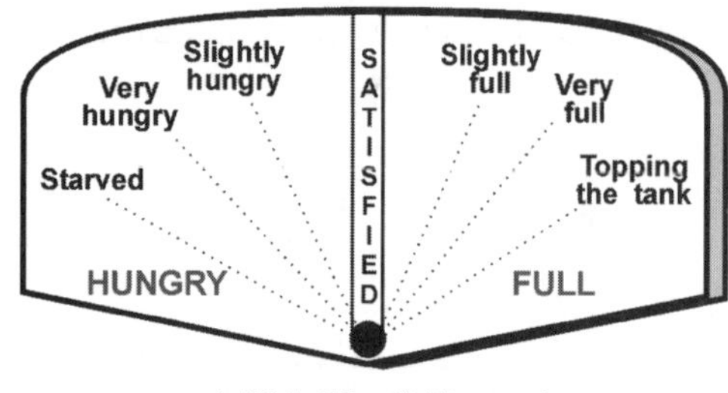

Hunger-fullness gauge.

There are different levels of hunger and fullness. When you're *Slightly Hungry,* you may have a somewhat empty feeling, but not much more than that. *Very Hungry* means that others are also aware of your hunger—your stomach is growling and grumbling. If you're at the *Starved* stage, you may be dizzy or feeling faint.

On the other side of the gauge are the relative levels of fullness. When you're *Slightly Full,* there's a somewhat heavy feeling in your stomach and awareness that hunger has already been taken care of many bites ago. *Very Full* is where you're starting to get uncomfortable, having a sensation of a very-stretched stomach. By the time you reach *Topping the Tank,* you've really overdone it. It's the same feeling you have on Thanksgiving, when you feel you just can't budge, where breathing is a little harder and you definitely are feeling gastric distress.

> Unless you're hungry (somewhere on the left side of the gauge), you shouldn't be eating. Let me say that again. If you're not hungry, you should not eat. That's a rule you should write in concrete, because that's what this plan is all about.

Notice that right in the middle of the two sides of the gauge is an area called "Satisfied." At this spot on the gauge, you're neither hungry nor full. You're feeling just right. That's the target range you're shooting for.

There's a problem with starting to eat when you're in the Satisfied range. You inevitably end up on the Full side of the gauge. The way this gauge is created, and the way you should think about eating, is that you should never end up in the Full range. Satisfied is as far as you should go. By eating into the Full range, you're consuming more food than your body needs. Remember, Satisfied is where you should be!

So at what point should you start eating? Eating when you get to Slightly Hungry is the best place, because you probably won't need to eat much to arrive back at Satisfied.

If you wait until Very Hungry or Starved, you're asking for trouble. Your choice of foods might not be as healthy. You might eat the first thing you see, even if it's not the best for you. Why do you think fast-food restaurants do so well? They cater to those who need food quickly, no matter whether it's the best choice or not.

Determining the "Satisfied" Level

What will it take for you to realize that you're at the *Satisfied* level after you've started eating? If there's no true bodily sensation as you'd have with being full (stomach stretched, feeling drowsy, uncomfortable), then how do you know when to stop? One of the first steps in this plan requires that you have your undivided attention on the eating process. There's no way you can recognize being satisfied if your mind is elsewhere. Watching television or reading a book is too much of a distraction to keep you focused.

Next, you need to do what you can to slow down your eating process. Remember, you need at least 20 minutes for food to send signals to your brain. After each bite, try to sense whether you've reached the Satisfied level (contented but not heavy or stretched feeling). One very clever way to slow yourself down is to eat your meal with the opposite hand from the one you normally use. After dropping food in your lap once or twice because of trying to keep up with your usual pace, you'll have to slow down. You could also use a smaller fork or spoon, such as a cocktail fork or baby spoon. Try putting your fork down between bites and asking yourself the question, "Have I had enough yet?"

You could try something my dog tends to do. He eats about half of what's in his bowl, then he walks around before coming back to finish. Sometimes he doesn't finish because he's full. You could take a quick "walkabout" after eating half of your meal or after 20 minutes has passed. When you return, ask yourself if you really want any more.

For those of you who want to use the gauge as a tracking device for when you start eating and when you have stopped, I've included a page of them in Appendix F.

Breakfast—the Meal of Champions

The alarm rings, but you're not quite ready to get up. So you push the snooze button, not just once but twice. By the time you make it out of bed, you realize that all you've got is 30 minutes to get dressed and eat breakfast. Obviously you have to get dressed. But that doesn't leave enough time for breakfast. So you tell yourself you'll grab something at break time from the vending machine.

Whoa! Let's rethink this. You're planning on passing up the most important meal of the day? You haven't fed your body anything since dinner last night. For some, that could be more than 12 hours ago. You may remember what I said in Chapters 11 and 12: Your liver only has so much glucose stored away. It's been using some of it during the night. What are you going to do to replenish its stores this morning? If you want your brain to work at peak performance, it would appreciate a little nourishment, thank you. During the night, your body has been in the "starving mode," using your energy stores to help you breathe, to help your heart beat and push blood around, to keep you warm, and so on. Now you plan to run off to work with nothing (and still expect your body to work on your behalf when your metabolism hasn't gotten a jump-start yet)?

If you ignore the hunger signals now, what kinds of healthy choices do you think you're going to make when everyone at work hears the grumbling sounds of your stomach emanating from your office? That's setting you up for a grab-and-run eating event. (And someone in the office always seems to be nice enough to bring in something sweet you can eat.)

Let's rewind the tape and you're back in bed. You have a choice to make. Do you push the snooze button or get up? If you want to perform well today, I'd suggest you eat breakfast. You may think that the extra minutes of snoozing will do you more good. They won't, because it's nutrition your body runs on. (This isn't to put down a good night's sleep because without that you're not going to perform at your peak. Maybe it means going to bed 10 or 15 minutes earlier, equivalent to the amount of time you expect from using the snooze button for in the morning.) It's no different from not putting gas in your car. It isn't going to get you to work on "empty." So let's think what would make for a good breakfast, both for one you sit down to and one you have ready to go for those mornings when you've cut it too close.

Fruit juice or cut-up fruit is a great start. Let's follow that up with some protein and carbohydrates. How about a scrambled egg and bran muffin, or a turkey sandwich on whole-wheat toast with a little bit of low-fat cream cheese and cranberry relish? Have a cup of hot chocolate on the side. (Make it with an artificial sweetener to decrease the calories.) Maybe there's something left over from dinner last night. Or you could make your own breakfast sandwich like some of the fast-food restaurants, using an English muffin and scrambled eggs. If you're trying to cut down on your cholesterol intake, use an egg substitute. If you don't want any preparation, try a bowl of granola or bran cereal topped with sliced bananas, sunflower seeds, and milk. If you don't like the idea of cooking breakfast in the morning, why not prepare it the night before? You could make a big pot of hot cereal and refrigerate it. Then in the morning, spoon out how much you want, heat it in the microwave, and top with dried cherries, slivered almonds, and low-fat cottage cheese. You've got a meal-in-a-bowl. Make a breakfast sandwich the night before and warm it in the microwave. I like the idea of making a big batch of whole-wheat pancakes on the weekend and freezing them. Pull out one or two the night before for breakfast and defrost in the microwave. Then roll up around a slice of ham and cheese. For another filling, you could spread some low-fat cream cheese on the pancake, a small amount of orange-flavored honey, and the ham. At least, if you don't have time to sit down to breakfast, you've got some healthy eating to take with you.

I think it first comes down to your appreciating the value of breakfast. It is given very little respect for the big job it has to do. I have to admit that sometimes when I get up early, I don't think that my stomach got up with me. I'm just not hungry. This is one of those times when I would have you go against the "eat only when you're hungry" rule. In most cases, I want you to respond to your body's signals, not those of your mind. However, in this case, there are enough studies to show the benefits of breakfast. Those studies also show that without it, you set yourself up for binging and actually being hungry the rest of the day. It's almost like your body is playing catch-up for not having gotten to eat in the morning.

Food Choices Still Matter

As much as I want you to learn to eat only to your Satisfied level and only when you're hungry, I still want you to eat healthfully. You could eat just enough doughnuts (make those Krispy Kremes!) to reach that level, but it wouldn't be nutritious. As I've suggested with other plans, I want you to read the Choice Plan. It gives you the best structure for a healthy diet. You get an idea of the number of servings from each food group that is right for your calorie level. Even if you don't like the structure that is part of that plan, just keep in mind what it means to choose healthfully when making your food selection in this R-U-Hungry Plan.

Fill 'Er Up

When trying to lose weight, many people fear they'll be hungry all the time. For some, the fear of hunger makes them eat more at each sitting as insurance for later. They also eat more often so as never to experience the pangs of hunger. Actually, experiencing hunger is a valuable thing because it tells us when we're in need of refueling. If you never get a sensation of hunger, you may always be in the mode of "Topping the Tank" when food really isn't necessary at that moment. I can offer you a way to eat that helps you fill up with less calories and that lasts longer.

The idea is to select foods that will both satisfy your appetite and control your eating for the same number of calories as foods that don't. Remember, losing weight is a matter of balancing calories taken in and calories burned. These foods I'm referring to have a greater amount of fiber, water, even air, to help you feel full. For example, you can eat 1 medium-size carrot for 30 calories. For that same 30 calories, you get only 2 potato chips. (When was the last time you were able to stop at two?)

The types of food that will fill you up and cost you fewer calories are fruits, vegetables, skim milk, nonfat cottage cheese, and broth-based soups. On the other end of the spectrum are the foods that are high in calories, such as cookies, chocolate candy, chips, nuts, and fats. These foods are going to cost us more calories and possibly not fill us up, calorie for calorie, as will the foods with plenty of fiber, water, or air. Sugar is an interesting food because of its effect on insulin. As I've discussed earlier in the book, the presence of sugar in your food stimulates the secretion of insulin, which in turn can cause a drop in blood sugar. This requires you to quickly "fill 'er up again." If you want the pleasure of getting to eat freely of foods without guilt, go for the lower-calorie choices that aren't loaded with sugar. Appreciate that a bigger volume of food in your stomach makes you feel more satisfied. High-fiber foods do this for you and cost you fewer calories. The brain is alerted that food is on the way. The more bulk there is in the food you eat, the longer it will take to digest and be absorbed, acting somewhat like a time-released satiety capsule.

Emotional Eating

True hunger is physiological. Your body needs energy and sends the signals to get you to eat. However, people will sometimes say that they're hungry in order to use food as a way of dealing with their emotions. It may harken back to our childhood days, when Mom gave us a cookie if we fell down or when a friend took away our favorite toy. Anger, frustration, and boredom should not be dealt with by eating. We're now adults and must learn to avoid using food as a Band-Aid for our problems.

In most cases, emotional eating doesn't involve true sensations of hunger. (There are some people who have ulcers or an excess production of stomach acids when they're upset; this may mimic the feeling of being hungry.) Really, our emotions are what need feeding. If you don't feed your emotions with food, then with what shall you feed them? You could talk over your problem with someone. "Getting it off your chest" might help. Maybe you could start a project that will divert your attention. Exercise is a healthy alternative. The scope of this book doesn't allow for any in-depth discussion of the psychological aspects of eating. If you know that emotional eating is your problem, seek counseling before overeating jeopardizes your health.

chapter 20

The Choice Plan

My mother's menu consisted of two choices:
Take it or leave it.
—*Buddy Hackett*

The *Balanced* Choice Plan is based on the recommendations of the American Heart Association, the American Dietetic Association, and the American Cancer Society. Being a balanced plan, it provides you with 55 percent of your calories from carbohydrates, 15 percent of calories from protein, and 30 percent of calories from fat. With this plan, you make food choices from each of the food groups shown on the Boomer's Guide Pyramid introduced in Part 1.

I'm also including a *Higher-Protein* Choice Plan for those of you who might be experiencing *insulin resistance.* Remember what I said in Chapter 12: Being overweight can set a person up for insulin resistance, and eating too many carbohydrates can exacerbate the problem. Your blood sugar level should be an indication. Have you had it tested lately? Because I believe that the risks of too much protein outweigh the benefits of eating the amount normally suggested on high-protein diets, I'm proposing here a blending of the balanced and the high-protein approaches. The *Higher-Protein* Choice Plan provides you with 20 to 25 percent of your calories from protein, 45 percent from carbohydrates, and 30 to 35 percent from fat.

I've included Sweets on the *Balanced* Choice Plan, and here's why: I'm hoping that if you like this plan, it will become your lifetime approach to eating. Now, if you like sweets, it doesn't make much sense to remove them on a permanent basis. I don't want you to consider them forbidden foods so that you crave them to the point of sneaking them or binging on them. It will be your decision whether you want to have them. Because they are a treat and not a requirement, you can save some calories by not eating them every day.

On the other hand, when you're on the *Higher-Protein* Choice Plan, you just don't have enough carbohydrate calories to spare on simple sugars. The point of being on this plan is so you don't get insulin spikes from excess carbohydrates, especially simple sugars. If you really feel that life won't be worth the living without having a sweet once in a while, let me suggest that you do the *Balanced* Choice Plan once a week and give yourself the treat on that day.

If you're a Planner, this is the perfect plan. It gives you a certain amount of organization, along with allowing you some freedom to make your own food choices. If you're the type who wouldn't mind keeping a food diary, you'll find this method even easier than the food diary. As I've mentioned in the discussion of the other plans, Ad-libbers, read this plan thoroughly, even if you don't want to follow it. It will give you some good background on which to make your eating decisions.

It's So Easy

The beauty of this plan is that "one choice" or serving from a food group has the same number of calories, grams of carbohydrates, protein, and fat as another choice from the same group. For example, one slice of bread has the equivalent nutrients as 3/4 cups rice. Each of these is equal to one Starch choice. You can swap one food for another within a group, and know that you're eating about the same number of calories and nutrients.

Think of this plan in terms of a savings account. The amount you have in your "food savings account" is equivalent to the number of choices you're allowed for each group every day. As you eat, you're taking a certain number of choices out of your savings account. By the end of the day, you'll probably have few or no choices left. Even though you've cleaned out your savings account of choices for the day, you get to start the next day with a new or fresh account. (Don't you wish your actual bank account worked that way?)

Your Daily Number of Choices

If you've decided on the *Balanced* Choice Plan, you must be wondering what your "savings account" amounts to. Here's how to find out. In Chapter 16, you determined how many calories is right for you in order to lose weight. Find on the *Balanced* Choice Plan in the following table the calorie level that is closest to that number of calories.

Run your finger along the row in the following table to see how many choices you get for each food category.

Number of Choices You Can Have on the Balanced Choice Plan

Calories	Starch	Veg	Fruit	Dry Beans/ Legumes	Milk	Meat	Fat	Sweets
1,200	4	4	2	1	1	3	4	1½
1,500	7	4	2	1	1	3	5	1½
1,800	8	5	3	1	1	4	6	1½
2,100	9	6	3	1	2	5	7	2
2,400	9	7	4	2	2	5	9	2

For example, someone on a 1,500-calorie plan would be allowed the following number of choices:

- 7 Starches
- 4 Vegetables
- 2 Fruits

- 1 Dry Beans/Legumes (1/2 cup per choice)
- 1 Milk
- 3 Meats (which means 3 ounces of a protein source)
- 5 Fats (1 teaspoon per choice; be sure you choose mono- and poly-unsaturated fats more often. Refer to Chapter 7 for examples of the different types of fat.)
- 1 1/2 Sweets

When you look through the food list in Appendix H, you'll see that if you select high-fat meats, you'll have to use up some of your allowances of Fat for the day along with your meat choices.

For those of you who want to try the *Higher-Protein* Choice Plan, the following table is where you'll find how many choices you get for the day.

Number of Choices You Can Have on the Higher-Protein Choice Plan

Calories	Starch	Veg	Fruit	Dry Beans/ Legumes	Milk	Meat	Fat
1,200	4	3	2	1	1	5	3
1,500	4	4	3	1	2	5	5
1,800	6	5	3	1	2	7	5
2,100	7	5	3	2	2	7	7
2,400	7	6	4	2	3	8	8

If your calorie level is higher than what's listed in either of the preceding tables, this is what I suggest. Combine two of the calorie levels that add up to your required calorie allowance. For example, if you determined that you should be eating 3,300 calories and you are going to do the *Balanced* Choice Plan, then combine the number of choices for the 1,500-calorie plan and the 1,800-calorie plan. Looking at the first table, you would be allowed the following:

- 15 Starches
- 9 Vegetables
- 5 Fruits

- 2 Dry Beans/Legumes
- 2 Milk
- 7 Meats
- 11 Fats
- 3 Sweets

Keeping Track of Your Choices

I don't know about you, but my memory isn't good enough to keep track of all the choices I eat during the day. That's why I created the Choice Tracker (see the following figure). The Tracker is set up for 1,500 calories on the *Balanced* Choice Plan and is partially filled in for the day. (There's a blank Choice Tracker in Appendix G, which you may copy for your own use.)

Setting up the Choice Tracker takes just a moment. Simply draw a line under the number of choices you're allowed for each food group. You just found out the numbers to use from the preceding tables. As you can see from the example, someone on 1,500 calories *Balanced* Choice Plan can have 7 Starches, so a line is drawn under the seventh circle in the Starch column. With 4 Vegetable choices, another line is drawn under the fourth triangle, and so on. For the Meat group, draw a line through all three columns and, lastly, draw a line under 5 Fats and 1½ Sweets. I'll be discussing those groups in more detail in a moment.

Did you notice on the Choice Tracker that there's a place for you to track your water intake? I've included that because people generally don't drink enough liquids. Hopefully, if you're tracking what you drink, you'll achieve the 8-glasses-a-day goal. You shouldn't wait for thirst to be your trigger. Some people don't experience a sense of thirst to know when it's time to start drinking.

I mentioned earlier that, for your own use, you can make copies of the Choice Tracker found in Appendix G. Let me recommend that you make a blank copy first. Then, on the blank Choice Tracker, draw the appropriate lines for your calorie level and the plan you've chosen to follow. Label the total number of calories in the space provided and the name of the plan. Now you can make copies of this submaster as you need them. That way you always have the master in the book, in case you need or want to change the calorie level or plan. By the way, if you choose to do the *Higher-Protein* Choice Plan, just scratch out the Sweets column (because you won't be using it).

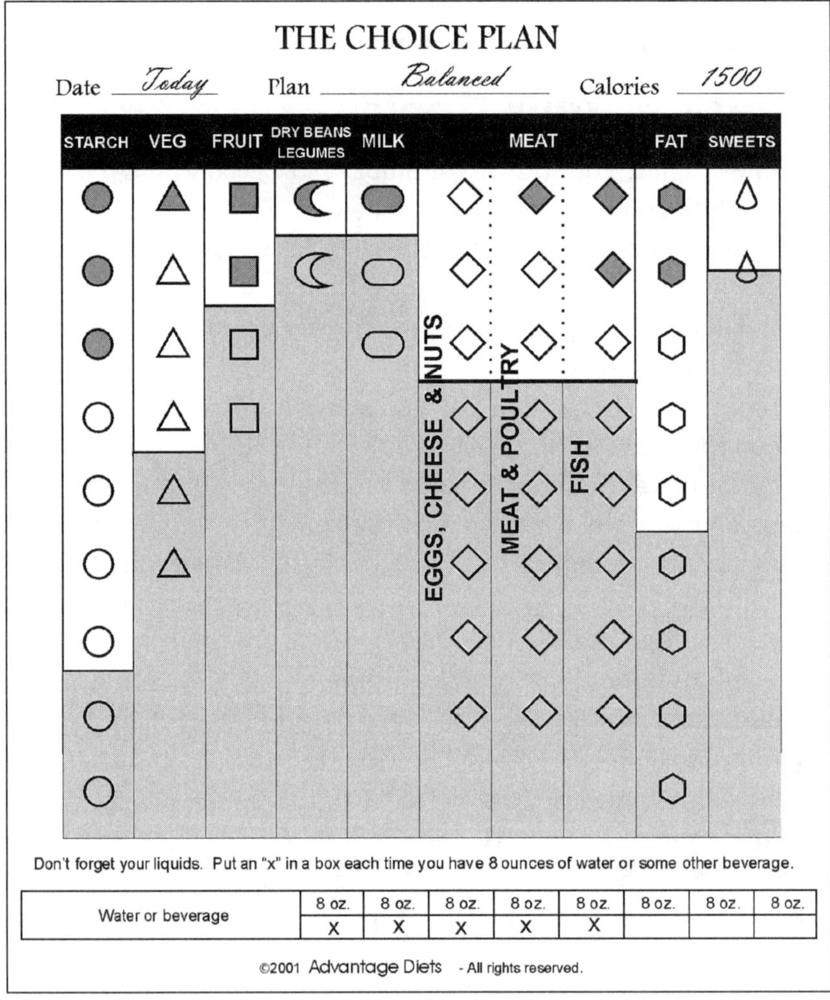

THE CHOICE PLAN

Date *Today* Plan *Balanced* Calories *1500*

STARCH | VEG | FRUIT | DRY BEANS LEGUMES | MILK | MEAT | FAT | SWEETS

EGGS, CHEESE & NUTS | MEAT & POULTRY | FISH

Don't forget your liquids. Put an "x" in a box each time you have 8 ounces of water or some other beverage.

Water or beverage	8 oz.	8 oz.	8 oz.	8 oz.	8 oz.	8 oz.	8 oz.	8 oz.
	X	X	X	X	X			

©2001 Advantage Diets - All rights reserved.

Choice Tracker for 1,500-calorie Balanced Choice Plan (partially filled in).

The white areas in the preceding figure show you the number of choices that someone eating 1,500 calories may have for each food group. Some of the choices have been filled in to show you how the Choice Tracker works.

For those of you eating more than 2,400 calories, use two trackers per day.

A Comment About Meat and Fat Choices

As you look at the Choice Tracker, notice that the meat group is divided into three columns:

- Eggs, Cheese, and Nuts
- Meat and Poultry
- Fish

Even though you drew a line under all those diamond shapes, **that doesn't mean you get to fill them all in.** Let me explain why the Choice Tracker is set up the way it is. Each diamond represents 1 ounce of food from the Meat group. You can select from any of the columns in the Meat group, having whatever combination of foods you want from that group. However, just limit yourself to the number of choices allowed for that group, based on your calorie plan. You should not have more of the diamond shapes colored in at the end of the day than the number of choices allowed at your calorie level.

For example, if you choose to eat 3 ounces of red meat (beef, pork, lamb, game, and so on) or poultry, you'd fill in 3 of the diamonds in the second column called Meats and Poultry. If you choose 1 ounce of nuts, 2 tablespoons of peanut butter, 1 egg, or 1 ounce of cheese, you'd fill in 1 diamond in the column Eggs, Cheese, and Nuts. (If you do select nuts, I suggest you limit yourself to 1 ounce. They may be a good source of protein, but they're high in fat.)

The same process applies for fish and seafood, which would be tracked in the last column, Fish.

As you can see from the sample Choice Tracker, the user filled in 1 ounce of poultry that she had for lunch and 2 ounces of fish for dinner.

For a 1,500-calorie plan, a total of 3 diamond shapes (or 3 ounces) is allowed for the *total* Meat group regardless of what type. The user just has to make sure that at the end of the day there aren't more than three diamond shapes filled in.

The reason for the different columns within the Meat group is to discourage you from relying solely on red meat for your meat choices. Fish is so healthy that research suggests eating one to two servings per week. When eating poultry, eat the breast meat, because it's lower in fat than other parts of the bird.

Although the fat group isn't divided into two columns, one for unsaturated fats (mono- and polyunsaturated) and the other for saturated fats (though I thought a long time about doing it that way), you need to really think about the kinds of fat you're eating. Remember my suggestions in Chapter 9. If you're going to eat from this group, you should consider having at least one to two servings of olive oil or another monounsaturated fat per day.

Let's Get Tracking

When you eat something, you'll be checking the food list in Appendix H for the values to use on your Choice Tracker. The following table is an example of what you'll find.

Food	Amt.	Starch	Veg.	Fruit	Beans/ Legumes	Milk	Meat	Fat	Sweets
Cereals and Grains									
Oats and oatmeal	½ cup	1							
Pasta, cooked	½ cup	1							
Puffed cereal	1½ cups	1							
Rice (white, brown), cooked	½ cup	1							

As you use up one choice from a food group, fill in the appropriate shape for that group on your Choice Tracker. For example, from the Food List you'll see that a ½-cup serving of rice is equal to 1 Starch choice. So you'd fill in one circle in the Starch column.

Of course, not all foods are as simple as a serving of rice. Maybe you want to eat something that combines several foods. For example, lasagna is made with noodles, tomato sauce, cheese, and meat. If you were to look up Lasagna with Meat in the Food List, you'd see the following:

It is very important that you take note of the serving sizes, which are listed under the Amt. column in the food list. Tracking for a 1/2-cup serving but eating 1 cup isn't going to help in your weight-loss efforts.

Food	Amt.	Starch	Veg.	Fruit	Beans/ Legumes	Milk	Meat	Fat	Sweets
Combination Dishes									
Lasagna with meat	1 cup	2	1½				2	2	

That tells you to fill in 2 Starch choices, 1½ Vegetable choices, 2 Meat choices, and 2 Fat choices. Because the meat in the lasagna is ground beef, you'd fill in two of the diamond shapes in the Meat and Poultry column.

If you're eating something that isn't listed in the food list, think about what the dish is made with and log each of the ingredients separately. Don't think that because you can't find the dish or don't know its exact ingredients, you needn't do any tracking. You're still eating the calories, so best you put something down (your best guess), or you're definitely going to go over your calorie allowance for the day. It may not show on the Choice Tracker, but it will definitely show on the bathroom scale.

Remember, after you've eaten up to the line you drew for your daily allowance of a particular food group, that's it. There's no more allowance for that group for the rest of the day. The more familiar you become with this system, the more planning you'll find yourself doing. This should keep you from going over your limit.

If you're finding that you're hungry, feel free to fill up on vegetables. Even though the table shows that you should have a certain number of vegetable choices for your calorie level, that guideline is more of a minimum than a maximum. Other than carrots and winter squashes, which have more sugar in them than most vegetables, vegetables are a good way to fill up but not out.

The reason that I like this system over such plans as calorie counting or counting fat grams is that it makes you aware of what food groups from which to eat. With those other systems, you could eat cake all day to fulfill your calorie or fat allowance, but never eat healthfully.

What About Packaged Foods?

It's unfortunate that the number of choices isn't listed on the food label. However, you could do some calculating on your own if you really want to. As I describe what to do with the information on a label, I'll be using the numbers found in the following table.

How Much Is in a Choice?

	1 Choice Has …			
	Calories	**Fat**	**Carbohydrates**	**Protein**
Starch	80	1 or fewer	15	3
Vegetable	25	0	5	2
Fruit	60	0	15	0
Milk (nonfat)	90	Trace	12	8
Meat (medium fat)	75	5	0	7
Fat	45	5	0	0

Note: Other than calories, values for the nutrients are in grams.

Let's say you're looking at a package of muffins. (Keep in mind that muffins are part of the Starch group.) Check out the Nutrient Facts on the label. The package I'm looking at shows the muffins having 146 calories, 6 grams of Total Fat, 20 grams of Carbohydrates, and 3 grams of Protein. From the following table, you can see that one muffin is at least one Starch choice (based on the information in the preceding table). With that 1 Starch choice, you've used up 80 calories, about 1 gram of fat, 15 grams of carbohydrates, and 3 grams of protein.

Interpreting the Label

	Label for Muffin Shows	1 Starch Choice Has	What's Remaining
Calories	146	80	66
Fat	6 g	1 g	5 g
Carbohydrates	20 g	15 g	5 g
Protein	3 g	3 g	0 g

Now what do you do with the remaining calories, fat, and carbohydrates? If you check out what a Fat choice is worth, you'd pretty much use up the remainder of calories and grams of fat. A Fat choice has 45 calories and 5 grams of fat. I wouldn't worry about the remaining 5 grams of carbohydrates. So on the Choice Tracker, you would color in one Starch choice and one Fat choice.

	Label for Muffin Shows	1 Starch Choice Has	What's Remaining	1 Fat Choice Has	What's Remaining
Calories	146	80	66	45	21
Fat	6 g	1 g	5 g	5 g	0 g
Carbohydrates	20 g	15 g	5 g	0 g	5 g
Protein	3 g	3 g	0 g	0 g	0 g

Sometimes when the food isn't clearly from one food group, as was true of the muffins, you need to consider the ingredients. That should help you assign the calories and amounts of nutrients to the various food groups. Consider, for example, a piece of pepperoni pizza: Some of the calories come from the dough, which is part of the Starch group; the tomato sauce and mushrooms are part of the Vegetable group; and the pepperoni and cheese are part of the Meat and Fat groups. If you were thinking about eating a slice, you would have to take some guesses as to how many of the calories and nutrients go to each choice within a group. However, you could apply the same approach we used with the muffins. It wouldn't be exact, but at least you'd get a general idea of how you were using up your calories and choices. As consumers, perhaps we can push the government to require food manufacturers to include information like this on the label.

chapter 21

The Choice Plan with Meal Planner

Most of life is choices, and the rest is pure dumb luck.
—Marian Erickson

The Choice Plan with Meal Planner is for the more structured Planner. It helps you plan exactly how many food choices should be eaten and when. Not only does it help set limits for each time you eat, it's also a way to prevent hunger getting the better of you. That's because you're eating frequently. By never getting really hungry, you don't run the risk of grabbing any food just to get rid of the hunger pains. You can make good, healthy decisions.

The Choice Tracker is set up slightly differently when you use it as a Meal Planner, as you can see in the following figure. Instead of just drawing a line under your daily allowance for each food category, you'll be drawing lines under the number of choices for *each meal*. You may find it helpful to write in the name of the meal, as shown in the example. As I suggested before, make a blank copy of the Choice Tracker. Then draw in your lines and names of meals. Use this as your submaster for multiple copies.

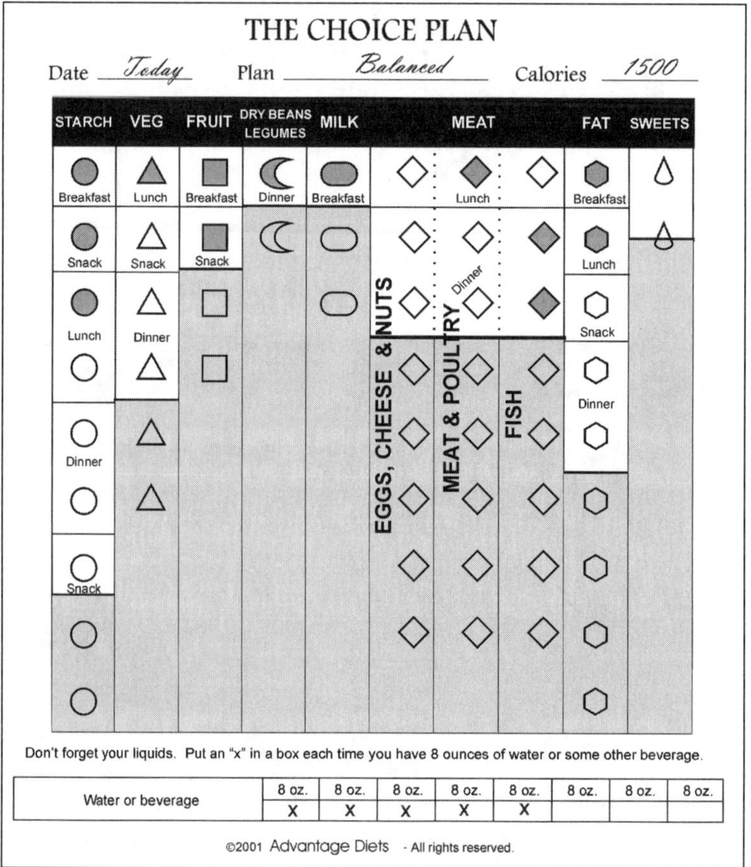
THE CHOICE PLAN

Date *Today* Plan *Balanced* Calories *1500*

STARCH | VEG | FRUIT | DRY BEANS LEGUMES | MILK | MEAT | FAT | SWEETS

Starch: Breakfast, Snack, Lunch, Dinner, Snack
Veg: Lunch, Snack, Dinner
Fruit: Breakfast, Snack
Dry Beans Legumes: Dinner
Milk: Breakfast
Meat: Lunch, Dinner — EGGS, CHEESE & NUTS; MEAT & POULTRY; FISH
Fat: Breakfast, Lunch, Snack, Dinner

Don't forget your liquids. Put an "x" in a box each time you have 8 ounces of water or some other beverage.

Water or beverage	8 oz.	8 oz.	8 oz.	8 oz.	8 oz.	8 oz.	8 oz.	8 oz.
	X	X	X	X	X			

©2001 Advantage Diets - All rights reserved.

Choice Tracker with Meal Planner for a 1,500-calorie Balanced Choice Plan.

Meal Planner for the *Balanced* Choice Plan

The following tables show you how to allocate your allowance of choices for meals and snacks on the *Balanced* Choice Plan. Find your calorie level and the meal suggestions I've made. Remember that these are just suggestions, so feel free to distribute your choices in a way that works for you. Sometimes when you see fat for a snack, what I had in mind was putting, for example, some cream cheese (Fat group) on celery sticks (Vegetable group) or on a bagel (Starch group).

Meal	Starch	Veg	Fruit	Dry Beans/ Legumes	Milk	Meat	Fat	Sweets
				1,200 Calories				
Breakfast	1	1		1		1		1½
Lunch	2	1				1	1	You decide
Snack		1	1				1	when you'd
Dinner	1	2		1		2	1	like it.
				1,500 Calories				
Breakfast	2		1		1		1	1½
Snack	1						1	You decide
Lunch	2	1	1			1	1	when you'd
Snack	1	1						like it.
Dinner	1	2		1		2	2	
				1,800 Calories				
Breakfast	2		1		1		2	1½
Snack	1						1	You decide
Lunch	2	2	1			2	1	when you'd
Snack	1	1						like it.
Dinner	1	2	1	1		2	2	
Snack	1							
				2,100 Calories				
Breakfast	2		1		1		2	2
Snack	1						1	You decide
Lunch	2	2	1			2	1	when you'd
Snack	1	2			1		1	like it.
Dinner	2	2	1	1		3	2	
Snack	1							
				2,400 Calories				
Breakfast	2		1		1		2	2
Snack	1						1	You decide
Lunch	2	2	1			2	2	when you'd
Snack	1	2			1		1	like it.
Dinner	2	3	1	2		3	2	
Snack	1		1				1	

Eventually, you may not even need the Tracker. However, I recommend that you use it for at least a month, if not longer. After a while, you should start thinking in terms of "Have I had my vegetable allowance for the day?" "Did I limit sweets or did I overdo it?" When you're finally doing that, you'll know you've adopted this approach as your lifetime way to eat. If you ever find yourself falling back into your old habits, pick up the Choice Tracker and start the procedure again. All you may need is a little refresher now and then to stay on course.

A Sample Meal Plan

To show you how to use the meal planner, let me share with you an example of what someone on 1,500 calories may choose to have.

- **Breakfast.** Fruit-flavored nonfat yogurt sweetened with artificial sweetener, topped with cereal and a banana
- **Snack.** Toasted bagel with cream cheese
- **Lunch.** Turkey sandwich with tomatoes and lettuce on whole wheat bread (topped with a drizzle of herb-flavored olive oil and vinegar) and sliced apple for dessert
- **Snack.** Medley of veggies with low-fat salad dressing dip
- **Dinner.** Spinach salad and garbanzo beans topped with basil-flavored olive oil and balsamic vinegar, grilled pork tenderloin, yam with margarine, and angel food cake for dessert.

Meal	Starch	Veg	Fruit	Dry Beans/ Legumes	Milk	Meat	Fat	Sweets
				1,500 Calories				
Breakfast	Cereal		1 small banana		3/4 cup artificially sweetened low-fat fruit-flavored yogurt			

Meal	Starch	Veg	Fruit	Dry Beans/ Legumes	Milk	Meat	Fat	Sweets
				1,500 Calories				
Snack	½ bagel						1 TB. cream cheese	
Lunch	2 slices whole-wheat bread	Sliced tomatoes and lettuce	1 small apple			1 ounce turkey	1 tsp. herb-flavored olive oil	
Snack		½ cup carrot, celery sticks, broccoli, string beans					1 TB. low-fat salad dressing	
Dinner	½ cup yams	2 cups raw spinach		½ cup garbanzo beans		3 ounces grilled pork tender-loin	2 tsp. olive oil 1 tsp. mar-garine	1 small slice angel food cake

Meal Planner for the *Higher-Protein* Choice Plan

Whenever you have some starch, be sure to have some protein, whether it comes from milk or meat, or you could include some fat with your starch. These additional foods will keep the starch from being absorbed too quickly and thereby control your blood sugar better.

Meal	Starch	Veg	Fruit	Dry Beans/ Legumes	Milk	Meat	Fat
				1,200 Calories			
Breakfast	1		1		1		1
Lunch	2	1				2	1
Snack		1	1				
Dinner	1	1		1		3	1

Meal	Starch	Veg	Fruit	Dry Beans/ Legumes	Milk	Meat	Fat
				1,500 Calories			
Breakfast	1		1		1		1
Lunch	2	2	1			2	2
Snack		1			1		
Dinner	1	1	1	1		3	2
				1,800 Calories			
Breakfast	1		1		1	1	1
Lunch	2	2	1			2	2
Snack	1	1				1	1
Dinner	1	2	1	1		3	1
Snack	1				1		
				2,100 Calories			
Breakfast	1		1		1	1	1
Snack	1						
Lunch	2	2	1			3	2
Snack		1	1				1
Dinner	2	2		2		3	2
Snack	1				1		1
				2,400 Calories			
Breakfast	1		1		1	1	1
Snack	1						1
Lunch	2	2	1			2	2
Snack		2	1		1		
Dinner	2	2	1	2		5	3
Snack	1				1		1

For Those Who Are Curious

Most people really don't know how much they eat during any given day. Diet studies show most people underestimate rather than overestimate how much they're eating. If you're curious about how much you're eating now before you embark on this plan, try this. Use the Choice

Tracker without drawing any lines as suggested previously. Leave the whole Tracker free to be filled in. (You may need two Trackers.) Then, for one week, fill in the shapes for the food groups that you eat from. Look at the food list in Appendix H for help. If you don't find the food you're eating, then select something similar or try to guess at the ingredients. No matter what, put something down. You ate it. It counts. At the end of the week (and not before), draw lines on these completed Trackers, showing the number of choices you will be allowed on your Choice Plan. How much more did you eat from the different food groups than your plan will permit? You should be able to see which food groups have been contributing the most calories. It's something you should keep an eye on, because those will be the food groups that might inch their way up in quantity when you're at the point of not using the Tracker on a daily basis.

Another bit of information you might want to know is the number of calories you've been eating. So here's something else you can do with the Choice Tracker you filled in. Multiply the total number of choices for each food group by the following numbers in the following table. Then add up your total to get the total number of calories for the day.

Food Group	Multiply By
Starch	80
Vegetable	25
Fruit	60
Dry beans/legumes	100
Milk (nonfat)	90
Meat (medium fat)	75
Fat	45
Sweets	75

chapter 22

Going Vegetarian

I was a vegetarian until I started leaning toward the sunlight.

—Rita Rudner

Vegetarianism has existed for centuries. In the mid-1800s, the Seventh-Day Adventists, viewing the body as a holy shrine, felt care should be given to it through healthy living. Tobacco and alcohol were forbidden, as was meat. Even cave dwellers thousands of years ago were vegetarians periodically when they had no success on a kill. In the 1970s, many boomers made it part of who they were as a generation. Vegetarianism encompassed their rebellion against the establishment and its meat-loving ways. Hippies, with their concern about pollution, wanted to protect the environment. Growing foods naturally and organically fit into this more perfect-world image. They believed that growing vegetables didn't rape the land the way raising cattle did. Hippies were for love and peace, not killing innocent animals. The idea of applying chemical fertilizers or pesticides to plants was, to them, against everything that nature originally intended. Refining foods was just as bad. They felt we should work responsibly with our environment to sustain it and ourselves. Bread, the staple of life, should be made from whole grains and should be hearty and crusty. The hippies started many of the farmers' markets that began to spring up in the 1980s. It was a place where they could sell their organically grown produce, fresh breads, and jams. Those who were part of the establishment may have found some of the hippies a little strange, but they still visited the farmers' markets for a pleasant afternoon and for good food.

Besides farmers' markets, co-ops were started in the 1970s. People could now buy in bulk. Whole foods played a large role. Foods grown locally from smaller farms became even more popular as a response to the "big guys," who had turned to hybridized produce that could be grown quickly, yield a mighty abundance, and be easily shipped to market with little destruction. With the population booming, I suppose I understand why farming practices took the turn they did. However, I believe flavor has been sacrificed for productivity. Has nutritional quality gone out the same door? I longingly remember when I was younger, eating carrots that actually were sweet. Today it's hard to find a decent carrot. Either we buy the organically grown produce in the market and pay top dollar for it or we plant our own. During World War II, our parents had planted "victory gardens." But after the war, when families started to become affluent, people preferred to spend their leisure time on more fun pursuits and leave the planting to the farmers.

The Many Faces of Vegetarianism

What is a vegetarian? The easy answer is it's a person who doesn't eat meat. Then it gets more complicated. There are the *lacto-vegetarians* who rely on dairy products as their main source of protein. The *ovo-vegetarians* incorporate eggs in their diet for protein. Put those two together and you have the *lacto-ovo-vegetarians,* people who incorporate both dairy and eggs in their diet. A *semi-vegetarian* is someone who will include fish or poultry, along with dairy and eggs, but avoids red meat. *Vegans* do not eat any animal protein, a diet practiced by such celebrities as Ben Affleck, Drew Barrymore, and Alicia Silverstone. Because animal products are the only food source of vitamin B_{12}, vegans must take supplements of the vitamin or eat plenty of foods that are fortified with it. Gwyneth Paltrow and Madonna have made the macrobiotic diet very popular. It, too, shuns meat, but views what we eat as only one branch of a many-branched tree of life. How we interact with our environment and the life we lead is an integral part of our health. What we're seeing today with vegetarianism harkens back to the days of the hippies, except it has now become mainstream.

When we hear about outbreaks of bacterial-borne illnesses due to eating meat, it's surprising that we all haven't gone vegetarian. Probably one of the most catastrophic outbreaks occurred in Washington State in 1993 when 741 people were infected with the E. coli o157:H7 bacteria found in undercooked contaminated ground beef at a fast-food restaurant. These people suffered bloody or severe diarrhea and dehydration. A young child died from complications. However, on the flip side, there was a recent news story that recommended avoiding alfalfa sprouts because they can have E. coli on them.

E. coli bacteria naturally exist in the intestines of cows. During the slaughtering process, if the intestines are cut, the bacteria can get onto the surface of the meat. Because a steak is a solid chunk of meat, the bacteria will only appear on the surface. Thoroughly cooking a steak on the outside should kill them off. Ground beef, on the other hand, has had the bacteria from the surface of the meat ground up and distributed throughout the meat. Therefore, it's essential that if you eat hamburger, you cook it through-and-through, getting the heat into the center of the patty. No more rare hamburger or, worse yet, Steak Tartar (raw hamburger).

Just because a small percentage of people have been affected by bacterial-borne illnesses in meats should not be your major reason for becoming a vegetarian. However, endorsing vegetarianism, or even semi-vegetarianism, because of its emphasis on plant foods is a healthy idea. It's a diet that's rich in phytochemicals and can be low in calories, especially if it doesn't include a lot of processed foods, which tend to contain a great deal of fat. With that said, you'd think that all vegetarians would be slim. That's not always the case, especially depending upon what kind of vegetarian they are. Lacto-ovo-vegetarians eat a lot of nuts and cheeses as their source of protein. The problem is that both of these foods are high in fat and calories. Because lacto-ovo-vegetarians assume vegetarianism is a healthy way to eat, they mistakenly eat freely of foods that can make them fat.

A Different Mind-Set

I find it interesting that people who want to be vegetarians often want food products that look like and taste like their meat counterparts. Someone expecting a veggie burger to taste like a hamburger is going to be pretty disappointed. Yet, a veggie burger enjoyed for its own qualities is a tasty dish. Veggie burgers made with soy are going to contain more protein than those made with rice. Check the label.

Years ago vegetarian food was boring. Now it has become a *cuisine*. If you're trying to switch over to being a vegetarian, you can still think in the same terms as a nonvegetarian, in that your plate should have sources of protein, starch, and vegetable. In fact, all of the diet plans you've read so far can be applied to vegetarian meals. It's just that your source of protein will be limited to eggs, dairy, poultry, and fish, with a heavy reliance on legumes and dry beans, for both their protein and starch content.

If you're looking for substitutes for dairy foods, consider soy milk, soy yogurt, soy margarine, and rice milk. Meat alternatives include meat analogs, tofu, tempeh, and wheat gluten. It's not that hard to put together a healthy and delicious vegetarian diet. For example, breakfast can consist of fruit, toast, hot chocolate, and a poached egg. Lunch could be pita stuffed with falafel, tahini sauce, sliced tomatoes, and sprouts. Finish the day off with a stir-fry dinner of tofu, veggies, and noodles, topped with nuts.

Besides feeling more environmentally responsible as a vegetarian, it's an overall healthier approach to eating and living. Because vegetarian diets tend to be low in saturated fat and cholesterol, they can help protect against heart disease. Being high in phytochemicals, vegetarian diets also can protect against cancer. Vegetarians also have a lower incidence of diabetes and hypertension.

Although vegetarians are eating in a healthy way, there's an accompanying mind-set of doing whatever else might be good for the body. You'll probably see many vegetarians doing yoga and meditation. They'll be into aromatherapy and massage. If they're taking supplements, they'll probably be herbal. Strict vegetarians think twice about what they're willing to put into their body. Caffeine and alcohol are normally restricted. The feeling is that, if it's not necessary for proper functioning, then why ingest it?

Getting Enough

Years ago there was a concern that vegetarians weren't eating a healthy diet. From the nonvegetarian perspective, vegetarians couldn't possibly be getting sufficient protein without eating meat. (Sometimes people forget that meat is not the only source of protein in our diet.) There are 20 different amino acids that make up the various proteins in our body. The human body makes all but nine of them. These nine are called "essential" because the body can't make them. Therefore, they must be provided by the diet.

The egg is considered the perfect or complete protein, because it has just the right balance of all the amino acids. Meat and fish come in as close seconds. But when the protein content of many other foods is analyzed, it's found that they're missing, or are somewhat deficient in, some of the amino acids. In 1971, Frances Moore Lappé, in her book *Diet for a Small Planet,* tried to show readers how they could mix complementary-protein foods, each incomplete unto itself, to make a more complete protein. For example, whereas dairy products have a good deal of the amino acid lysine, many nuts and seeds are deficient in that nutrient. So by mixing the two foods, one food's strength can make up for the other's deficiency. The accompanying figure shows you some of Lappé's suggestions for combining foods.

> *Should vegetarians eat animal crackers?*
>
> *—Jerry Seinfeld*

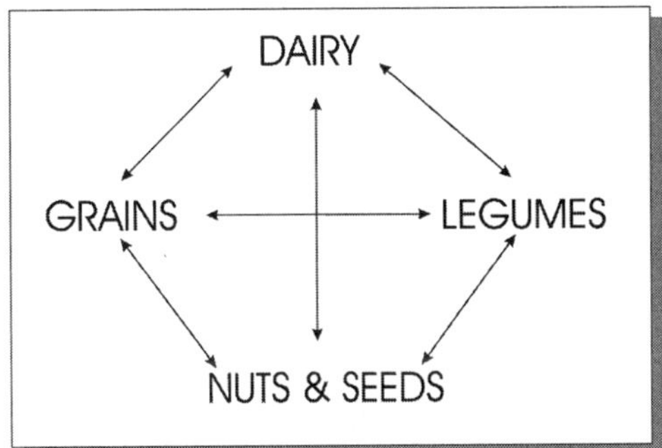

Complementary proteins.

At the time, it was recommended that you eat the complementary foods at the same time. That way, it was thought, the amino acids would be as nearly complete as possible when eaten. Over the years, we've learned that it isn't necessary to eat them at the same time. As long as sometime during the day the diet supplies all of those amino acids, the body will use them as necessary. (Remember, your body is a lot smarter than you give it credit for.) Of course, you may find menu planning easier if you consider the protein combinations. I can see having cheese and crackers or cereal and milk to satisfy the Dairy-Grains combination. Rice and lentils will give you your Legumes-Grains combination.

One mineral of concern for a vegetarian is iron. Plant foods contain a form of iron that's not as readily absorbed as iron from meat. Eating foods that are high in vitamin C along with high-iron plant foods will help improve the iron absorption. For example, spinach is high in iron. Having a spinach salad with orange segments would increase the chances that the iron from the spinach will be absorbed. Calcium is another mineral that only vegans—who don't drink or eat any milk products—should worry about. Fortunately, many vegetables, especially green leafy ones, contain calcium. Soy milk fortified with calcium and vitamin D would be a good idea. It wouldn't hurt, however, for vegans to take a calcium supplement, along with vitamin D for better calcium absorption. Getting some exposure to sunlight for a short time will also improve one's vitamin D status. Zinc is often hard for even nonvegetarians to get enough of, unless they're eating a sufficient amount of meat. Therefore, it would be a good idea for vegetarians to take a zinc supplement, unless they can get their zinc requirements from their foods.

Check out the following table for good sources of the various minerals that vegetarians might be deficient in. Even for nonvegetarians, it's good information to use for selecting foods. The foods in each category are listed in descending order of nutrient quantity per serving. A typical serving of legumes is 1/2 cup, cereal is 3/4 cup, milk is 1 cup, cheese is 1 ounce, vegetables is 1/2 cup cooked, juice is 3/4 cup, and nuts and seeds is 2 tablespoons.

Food Sources of Nutrients

Calcium	Iron	Zinc	Vitamin D	Vitamin B_{12}
Fruits:	**Breads, cereals, and grains:**	**Breads, cereals, and grains:**	**Breads, cereals, and grains:**	**Breads, cereals, and grains:**
Calcium-fortified orange juice	Bran flakes	Bran flakes	Fortified, ready-to-eat cereals	Ready-to-eat cereals
Dried figs	Oatmeal	Wheat germ	**Soy products:**	**Soy products:**
Legumes:	Cream of Wheat	Whole-wheat bread	Fortified soy milk	Meat analogs
Navy beans	Wheat germ	Whole-grain products		Fortified soy milk
Vegetarian baked beans	Whole-wheat bread	**Dairy products:**		Nutritional yeast
Great northern beans	**Fruits:**	Yogurt		
Black beans	Dried fruit	Cow's milk		
Pinto beans	Prune juice	Cheddar cheese		
Chickpeas	**Legumes:**	**Legumes:**		
Nuts and seeds:	Garbanzo beans	Adzuki beans		
Almond butter	Lentils	Chickpeas		
Almonds	Navy beans	Lentils		
Other foods:	Lima beans	Lima beans		
Yogurt	Black beans	**Nuts and seeds:**		
Cow's milk	**Nuts and seeds:**	Almonds		
Blackstrap molasses	Pumpkin seeds	Cashews		
Soy products:	Tahini (sesame seeds)	Peanuts		
Tofu—calcium processed	Sunflower seeds	**Other foods:**		
	Cashews			

Food Sources of Nutrients *(continued)*

Calcium	Iron	Zinc	Vitamin D	Vitamin B_{12}
Soymilk, fortified	**Other foods:**	Eggs		
Soy nuts	Blackstrap molasses	**Vegetables:**		
Soybeans	Egg yolks	Peas		
Tempeh	**Soy products:**	Corn		
Vegetables:	Tofu			
Collard greens	Soybeans			
Turnip greens	Soy milk			
Kale	Tempeh			
Bok choi	**Vegetables:**			
Mustard greens	Swiss chard			
	Turnip greens			
	Beet greens			
	Tomato juice			

part 4

Some Tools for Your Kit

Just as a carpenter needs a hammer and nails to do the job, you, too, need some tools to do your job of losing weight. Without the proper tools, you may not be as successful as you'd like. How many times have you needed a screwdriver and tried to manage the job with a kitchen knife? The screw may go part of the way into the hole, but getting it really tight is another story. Yet, had you gotten the screwdriver from the start, the job would have been done right. That's why, in these chapters, I share with you some of the tools I think will make your job easier—such as how to be savvy in the supermarket, knowing what to look for on a food label, learning ways to make cooking easy and fun, choosing healthy snacks, and how to dine out healthfully.

chapter 23

Supermarket Smarts

The odds of going to the store for a loaf of bread and coming out with only a loaf of bread are three billion to one.

—Erma Bombeck

Grocery shopping is something we all have to do on a regular basis, whether we eat all our meals at home or eat many of them out in restaurants. I don't know anyone who has a personal shopper. (However, I'm sure there are some who would love to have one. The website HomeGrocer.com tried to provide the service but wasn't successful and went out of business.) I'd like to make the process more enjoyable and ensure that you come out of the store with a bag full of healthy choices. Because there are many challenges to face in the grocery store, let me see if I can help.

The grocery stores that my mother shopped in were not nearly the size of today's supermarkets. Even though the supermarkets had all the food departments we have today, if you really wanted quality, you went to specialty stores. I can remember when I was a young girl, I'd go with my mother to the butcher shop, where all they sold was meat. You could get it trimmed the way you liked. Then there was the poultry shop where I watched the butcher actually burn the feathers off of the fresh birds. Produce stores were often smaller than the produce departments found in today's major supermarkets. It seemed back then people were willing to walk or drive from store to store, picking up their groceries. It could be an all-day affair. However, with more stay-at-home moms then, that was part of their job description. They developed friendships with the butcher or grocer, who knew you by name. Shopping wasn't just buying food; it was also an opportunity for chatting, catching up on the latest news.

In some ways, the arrival of the supermarket was a great boon. You could now get everything you needed in just one stop. The competition for your dollar became very keen. In fact, during the 1950s, many stores offered trading stamps to get your business. The most popular stamp was S&H Green Stamps (though others were Blue Chip, Top Value, and Gold Bond). You were given one S&H Green Stamp for every dime you spent. Then, when you had enough stamps, you'd put them in little booklets. It used to be a job given to us kids to lick all those stamps. After enough stamps had been collected, you could trade them in on merchandise through catalogs or at redemption centers. That program lasted only so long because it cost markets too much money to sponsor it. Some markets advertised that their products cost less because they didn't offer stamps and started getting the business that the stamps were supposed to promote.

With all the competition came more quantity, variety, and exotic choices. Food manufacturers have helped fill the shelves with things we need, as well as things we would be healthier without. Just remember that what you put in your cart is a matter of choice. If you're taking something home that you shouldn't be eating, remember who put it there.

Some Basic Rules of Shopping

Make a shopping list and take it with you. You know how frustrating it is to be in the grocery store, trying to remember what it was you needed. If only you had looked in the refrigerator and pantry before you left home, you'd know what to buy. If only you had planned a week's worth of menus and put them on a list, you'd be prepared for the week. Even better would be to have a list posted on the refrigerator that you could add to throughout the week before you went shopping.

Don't shop when you're hungry. You're just asking for trouble if you do. When you're hungry, you're less apt to walk past those product samples they're giving out. You may want to convince yourself that you're trying them just to decide whether you want to buy the product. Who are you fooling? Sometimes I think people buy the product because they feel guilty for eating the samples. If you time it right (around lunchtime or dinnertime), you could have quite a meal before you leave the store. Did you think that because you're eating while pushing your cart around the market those calories don't count? Or that because they seem like such small portions, what's the harm? Think again. Calories do add up. When we were growing up, we rarely got samples to try. Manufacturers hadn't yet discovered the promotional value. Sometimes I wonder if we were better off. There were at least a few less temptations to get in our way. Shopping on an empty stomach means it's going to be harder to stick to a grocery list (if you remembered to make one and bring it with you).

Shop alone. When my husband shops with me, we invariably go home with things that were not on the list. I must admit that I often enjoy the adventure of exploring the aisles for new foods. (Be careful—two sets of eyes see more than one set does!) Markets today offer such a wide array of foods that it seems a shame not to try them. Many of the unusual foods that have ended up coming home with us were tasty discoveries. However, if you're trying to stick to a budget and a calorie limit, it may be best to leave your loved ones at home. That includes the kids. Supermarkets are clever in their arrangement of foods. Have you ever noticed where they place the sugared cereals and chips? Yep, at kids' eye level. The television advertisers haven't helped us out here either. With all their promotion of various products, our kids get sucked in, while the dollars in our wallets get sucked out. Also, notice that the more

> How many times have you arrived at the cash register with more than you really needed, saying, "But I only came in for a gallon of milk"?

expensive items are placed at eye level, whereas the least expensive are on the lowest shelf.

Coupons may not be your best deal. If food manufacturers don't get your attention through television and magazine advertisements, they'll try to get it with coupons in the newspaper or in mailers. It seems like such a good deal. Twenty cents off this product or two-for-one on that product seems hard to pass up. How many coupons have you clipped out of the newspaper or saved from a mailer that were for a food you never eat, but was such a bargain? Of course, you may say that you took it out because you'd heard about it on television and here, lo and behold, was an opportunity to try it for less. Just be sure that you're buying it because you truly want it and not because the advertisers have done a good job of influencing you. The calories still count even if you didn't enjoy what you ate. Worse yet is eating certain foods because you don't want to waste them or the money you spent for them. You'd be better off giving them away.

Buying in quantity may or may not be the best deal. As is often the case, if you buy something in quantity, you'll pay less per item than when it comes in smaller packages. That's great if it's something you use frequently and regularly. However, if it's a perishable food that may go bad before you've been able to use it all, your good deal may go out the window. And if you try to eat it quickly enough to avoid spoilage, it's not going to help your weight management efforts. If you have a freezer or the storage space, then buying in quantity may help your budget. When we were growing up, warehouse stores such as Costco or Sam's Club didn't exist. Now we're provided with the opportunity to buy more for less. But that means you may have more temptations sitting around the house than if you bought foods in smaller packages. You need to ask yourself whether you can handle having so much available without having to answer the call to overeat. Another ploy by the grocery store that encourages people to buy more is having a sign that says, "3 for $3," rather than $1 each. It's the same thing but sells more. Don't get suckered in.

Stay away from the end-aisle displays. That's where the stores really get you. End-aisle displays rarely have the healthiest choices of foods. They tend to be more expensive, as well. There's no question that end-aisle displays get your attention—that's what they're designed to do. Now that I've warned you, keep that in mind the next time something from the end of an aisle ends up in your cart. Did you really want it? Watch out for special-tag items, as well. Unless those foods fit into the plan you've chosen to follow, no price should be considered low enough to entice you. Another thing to be wary of are those things called "impulse items" located at the check-out stand. Invariably, you'll have to wait in line to be rung up. That gives you plenty of time to look over the candy bars and other goodies the store has put there to tempt you. They're often in small enough packages to seem harmless. Resist! Pick up a magazine and start thumbing through it. It'll keep your hands busy and your mind off food. And just think of the latest gossip you'll get to read about (and you won't have to pay for the magazine).

Whereas we take it for granted that we can get everything from meat and produce to beauty products and kitchenware in our local markets, that wasn't the case before World War II. During World War II, grocery stores couldn't always stock their shelves with foods. With rationing, the shelves were often empty. So owners of grocery stores figured they might as well carry newspapers, magazines, beauty products, and kitchenware just to have something to sell.

Grocery Store Roadmap

If you want to find the healthiest foods in the market, walk around the perimeter of the store. Look at the following diagram (which is typical for most stores) and notice the location of the major food groups. Most of the unprocessed foods line the walls of the grocery store. It's the aisles in the middle of the store where the manufacturers can get the best of you. These days, with all the packaged frozen foods (and I'm not talking about the plain frozen vegetables!), the frozen-food section can be just as dangerous as the canned- or boxed-food aisles. The colorful and appealing packaging may tempt you. You may think, "What's the harm in stopping and looking? What is it? I wonder what it tastes like? Well, the only way to find out is to try it." As I said earlier, I'm all for exploring new foods. But you better read the label first. (We'll go over that in the next chapter.)

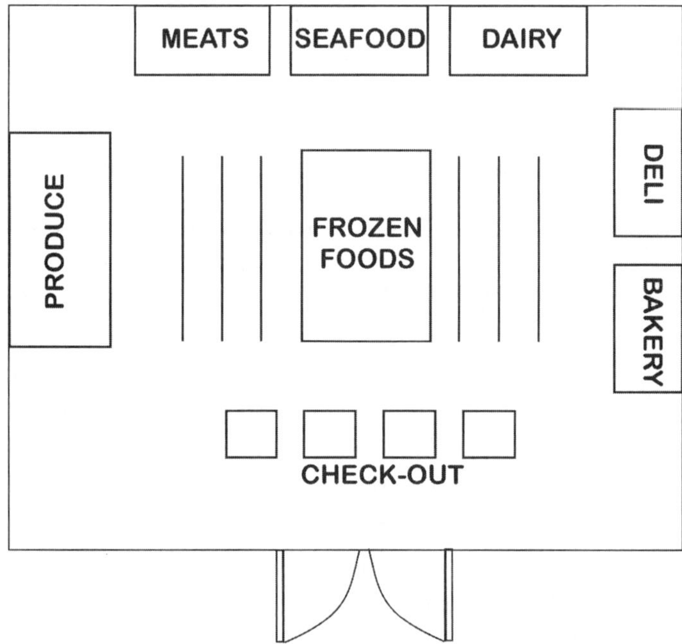

Typical grocery store layout.

Because the freezer section takes up so much space in a supermarket, let's spend a moment trying to determine how best to approach it. The vegetable section is easy if you stick with the plain vegetables. It's the vegetables in sauces where you need to think twice. You figured out your calorie allowance in Chapter 16. Is that sauce really worth spending some of your calorie allowance on? Are you willing to pass up something else because of it?

The entrées can definitely get you into trouble with so many of them being high in fat and calories. It's time for you to do some label reading. (I'll be sharing more about that in the next chapter.) When you know you're allowed so many calories per day, this entrée and whatever else you have for that meal shouldn't exceed more than one third of your total daily allowance for calories and fat. (It's less if you're dividing your day up with three meals and two snacks.) I don't want to set limits here, saying any entrée you select should have no more than so many calories and grams of fat. For each of you it will be different. You definitely need to have some idea when you're making the selection. Many of the entrées make the calculations and portion size easy for you; a package is often one serving. (Look closely. You just may have to share it with someone when it says "Number of Servings: 2.") Because the portion size is determined by the government, that doesn't necessarily mean you have to eat the whole thing if it won't fit into your calorie requirements or you're not hungry for it.

The area devoted to pizzas is the section in the freezer that can cause problems for people. First, you're talking about a high-fat food. Second, unless you take note of how many slices make up one serving, it won't matter what's on the label when you eat as much as you want. And even if you eat according to the package's serving size, you still have to consider how it fits into your calorie allowance.

The dessert section can pose nearly as many obstacles as the entrée section when it comes to selecting low-fat varieties. However, food manufacturers have provided many lighter versions of ice cream to satisfy your sweet tooth. Compare the high-fat and low-fat choices and see the value in selecting the low-fat choices more often. Also, don't be swayed by the individually wrapped frozen desserts. There is no law that says you have to finish the whole thing. It can be put back into your freezer for another time. Then there are frozen fruits, which are always a good choice for dessert.

You might want to check out the vegetarian foods even if you're not a vegetarian. Most of the selections are fairly low in fat and calories and high in fiber. Let me just warn you not to take home a package of veggie burgers, grill them, and expect them to taste like hamburger. They're delicious and healthful in their own right, but disappoint the eater who has expectations of beef. You can dress them up like a hamburger with the bun, tomato, lettuce, and ketchup, though. Even some of the vegetarian sausages or fake chicken aren't bad.

As you walk around the store, keep in mind what plan you're on as you make your selections. If it's the Choice Plan, then you will know how many choices you have available for a particular meal. If it's the Portion-Control Plan, then look at what the package says is a serving size. If it's the Instead Plan, compare foods to find the food with the lowest number of grams of fat and calories. If it's the R-U-Hungry Plan, then whatever you decide to buy, remember to eat it slowly so you can really sense when you've had enough. When food first arrives in your stomach, it doesn't know how many calories hit it. Remember what I shared in Chapter 19? The volume of the food rather than its calorie content has more impact in the beginning of the meal. So having a salad with low-fat dressing first before you start to eat the entrée will help keep you from overeating.

chapter 24

What's on the Label

We are living in a world today where lemonade is made from artificial flavors and furniture polish is made from real lemons.

—Alfred E. Newman

If you're a health-conscious consumer, take a little time to read labels. With so many foods from which to choose, the information on the label can help you make a healthy selection. Read the words on the front of the package and the nutrient information (Nutrition Facts) listed on the side or back of the package to learn the best choices.

When we were growing up, who read labels? Not that there was much to read anyway. At that time, the only information manufacturers had to display on the label was the name of the food, its net weight, and how to contact the manufacturer. Times definitely have changed. Now there is a whole wealth of information available to us. Since the 1940s, there's been a great deal of development in the look of the label and what manufacturers must include. By the 1970s, the Food and Drug Administration (FDA) had set up a voluntary nutrition labeling program. However, only fortified foods or foods that advertised health claims had to include some information about the nutrient content.

At the time, a favorite nutrient content claim to entice you to buy a product was "contains no cholesterol." Do you remember that? It seemed that products flew off the shelf if they could tout that the food contained no cholesterol. Of course, no one was telling you about how much fat was in the product, and that it's the total and saturated fat that can increase your risk of heart disease. They also weren't mentioning the fact that if a food contained no meat, it couldn't contain any cholesterol, because plant foods (such as grains, legumes, vegetables, fruits, and vegetable oils) don't have any. Potato chips sounded so healthy when we were told they didn't contain any cholesterol. But what about all that fat? Fortunately, there are tighter controls over what health claims can be made on labels today.

Are We Being Deceived?

The Nutrition Labeling and Education Act of 1990 was a landmark move by the government. The government now had the power to regulate what must appear on a label, as well as what couldn't be included. Even with these rules, food manufacturers didn't, and still don't, mind being deceptive if it'll help sell a product. Watch out for such phrases as "made with real ____" and "fruit juice added." In either case, you don't know how much is included, but are being led to believe that you're getting more than is probably there.

Another common deception is the picture on the package. The label may show an oven-toaster tart surrounded by fresh strawberries, as if all those strawberries were put into one of those tarts. You're lucky if you get even one or two strawberries. However, you are getting plenty of sugar and you're paying a high price for it. The size of the writing on the label may also influence you. The other day I was in the market and saw a package of fat-free crackers with the word *Vegetable* on the front, in lettering so large that it overpowered the rest of the writing. So I wondered just how many vegetables were in a serving. By reading the Nutrition Facts and the ingredient list, the answer I got was "not much."

And shame on the package designers who make the list of ingredients almost impossible to read. Many of us boomers have to wear glasses in order to read the fine print, which often needs even a magnifying glass to decipher. Why put the ingredients in such a small font size and a color that blends in so much with the background? It doesn't help to put all the words in capital letters with too little space between letters either. Don't the manufacturers really want us to know? I could go on, but I'm sure you get my point. So watch out for these deceptive practices. One way is to read the Nutrition Facts and ingredient list on the label (if you can make out the words). Keep in mind that ingredients are listed in descending order of weight. Whatever comes first in the list contributes the most to the food.

The job of the food manufacturer is to get you to buy their products. The package designers know what sells products. The color of the package can make a huge impression on a shopper. Black is a symbol of quality. Reds stimulate people's appetite. (Think about the color scheme of McDonald's.) Green makes people think the manufacturers care about the environment. (Remember Greenpeace?) It also makes consumers think that the products are healthier. (Look at the Healthy Choice line of foods.) Brown is an earthy color and makes people think the foods are baked or roasted and rich in flavor.

Let's take a closer look at a label, in the following figure, to understand how to select healthier food choices. The first thing you should look at is the **Serving Size** in section 1. It won't do you any good to know how much of any nutrient is in a serving if you don't know what the serving size is. You'd be amazed how many people miss this bit of information and eat far more than they should. A perfect example is granola cereal. How much do you think is a serving? If you've eaten flake cereals, you'd probably figure it to be about $\frac{1}{2}$ to 1 cup. However, granola is very dense and, in many cases, high calorie, so that a serving size of it is only about $\frac{1}{4}$ cup. Also, take special note of the **Servings per Container.** Some containers look as if they're packaged for one person. Take a closer look. Although a 6-ounce can of tuna would seem like about the right amount for 1 person (those cans look so small), its label says $2\frac{1}{2}$ servings.

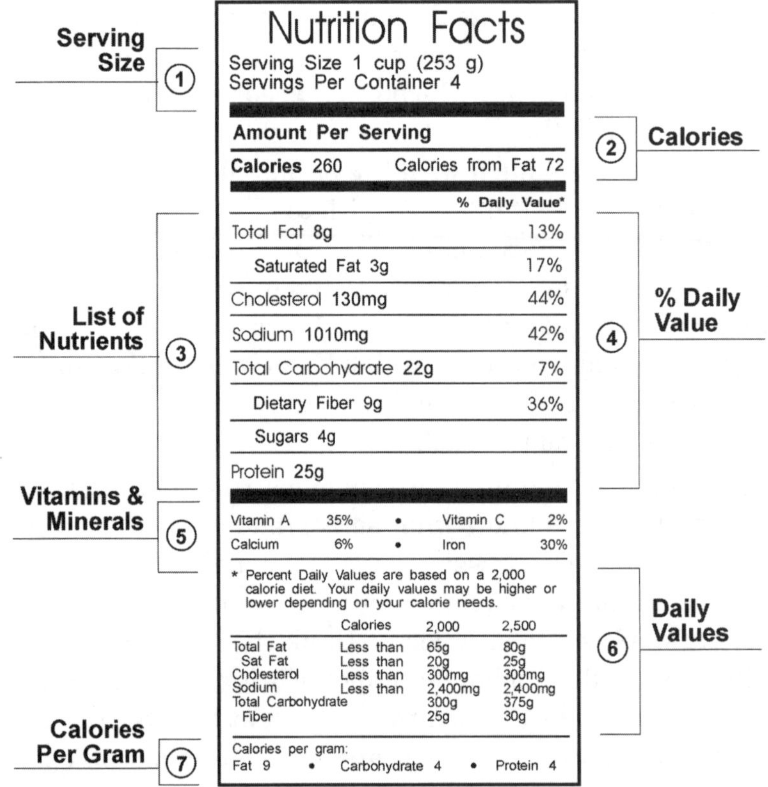

Food label for chili.

Section 2 provides total **Calories** per serving and **Calories from Fat.** With these two numbers, you could find what the percentage of fat is in the food. Let me save you the trouble. Years ago, people misinterpreted the guideline that stated we should eat no more than 30 percent of our calories from fat. They assumed that meant each food they ate had to contain less than 30 percent fat. (Some foods that require preparation—for example, adding eggs or fats—may list both the values for "as prepared" and "package mix," in case you make any changes to their suggestions.)

What that kind of thinking promoted was that any food with more than 30 percent fat was unhealthy. Olive oil, for example, which we know to be one of the healthy monounsaturated fats, would have to be eliminated from the diet. It's 100% fat. What's actually important is how your diet adds up for the day. That's why the FDA developed the concept of "**% Daily Value** (%DV)," which you can see in section 4.

%DVs represent an approach to nutrition information where you don't judge a food by its specific grams or milligrams of a nutrient. Rather, %DV is a way of looking at a food's nutrient contribution to the overall diet. The numbers in section 4 will serve as your guide. They show you how much of your day's allowance for a nutrient you use up when eating the food. From that, you can figure what you have left for the day. A quick example might help. A teaspoon of oil has a %DV of 8 percent. After eating a serving of the oil, you still have 92 percent of your daily fat allowance (DV) left to spend.

To understand %DV, you first must know about Daily Values. Daily Values (DVs) are the currently accepted nutrition recommendations set by the government. They are based on someone eating 2,000 calories a day, a level referred to as the *reference diet*. The FDA initially wanted to set the level at 2,300 calories, but many health professionals argued against it, stating it was too high a level for too many Americans. You may then wonder how you're supposed to use the label if you're not eating 2,000 calories. That's why I created the *% Daily Value Converter* that you'll find in Appendix I. You'll also find a table showing the *Daily Values for Different Calorie Levels*.

The DVs, which appear at the bottom of the label in section 6, are calculated as follows: Total fat is 30 percent of total calories, saturated fat is 10 percent of total calories, total carbohydrates is 60 percent of total calories, and fiber is 11.5 grams per 1,000 calories.

Here are some rules of thumb to remember as you read the label:

The 5% Rule: Look for %DV of less than or equal to 5% to get a *low source* of a nutrient. This rule comes in handy when you're trying to limit your fat intake.

The 20% Rule: When the %DV is greater than 20%, the food is considered a *high source* of a nutrient. That's great if you're looking for increasing your fiber intake, but it's something to watch out for when trying to decrease your fat intake.

Section 3 lists the grams or milligrams of each nutrient. Section 5 specifically includes the %DV for vitamins A and C, iron, and calcium because they're the nutrients that are most often deficient in the diet. Sections 6 and 7 give general information for interpreting the label values. This information is the same no matter what the product. Take note that 1 gram of fat contains 9 calories, 1 gram of carbohydrates contains 4 calories, and 1 gram of protein contains 4 calories. As you can see, 1 gram of fat is more energy dense than carbohydrates or protein. That's something to keep in mind when you're making food selections.

Label Lingo

Here are some terms to watch for:

- **Cholesterol-free food.** By including the word *food,* the claim means that the food is naturally free of cholesterol. Compare that to "cholesterol-free," showing that the food has been made without cholesterol.
- **Free.** For a particular nutrient, "free" is where there is none or only a trace amount. For sugar and sodium, that means fewer than 5 grams. For calories, "free" means fewer than 5 calories. For total fat and saturated fat, "free" means fewer than 0.5 grams. You may wonder how a product can say "0" grams of fat when you can see some fat listed under ingredients. That's because labels are allowed to round off to give a whole number. Because less than 0.5 grams rounds off to "0," the label can say "0" grams.
- **Good source/High source.** For a product to be a "good" source of a nutrient, it has to have between 10% and 19% of the DV for that nutrient. If it's a "high" source, those percentages go up to 20% and above. For example, if a container of orange juice states it is a "high source of vitamin C," it means that for 1 serving you're getting at least 12 milligrams of the vitamin. (The DV for vitamin C is 60 milligrams; therefore, 20% of 60 milligrams = 12 milligrams.)

- **Juice/beverage/drink/cocktail.** When a product says "juice," it means it is 100 percent real juice (for example, apple juice). However, when a product says "beverage," "drink," or "cocktail," it contains less than 100 percent real juice. In these cases, there's no way for you to know just how much juice you're getting, unless the manufacturer states it on the label. You could be getting a lot of water and sugar.
- **Lean.** This term is used for a 100-gram serving of meat, poultry, and seafood products, as well as main dish, meal, and meal-type products. Total fat must be fewer than 10 grams, saturated fat fewer than 4 grams, and cholesterol fewer than 95 milligrams.
- **Light or lite.** The product with this label must have one third fewer calories *or* 50 percent less fat than a standard reference serving (determined by the government).
- **Low.** If the term is referring to . . .

  Total fat, the product must have 3 grams or fewer of fat.

  Saturated fat must be 1 gram or fewer and no more than 15 percent of calories from saturated fat.

  Cholesterol has to be 20 milligrams or less, and the product can't contain more than 2 grams of saturated fat.

  When the label is referring to *sodium,* the food cannot contain more than 140 milligrams of sodium.

  A product called low calorie cannot have more than 40 calories.
- **Reduced.** This means that the manufacturer has reformulated the food product so it has less of certain nutrients than the regular or reference product. However, the food may still contain large amounts of certain nutrients. The major point here is that the food contains at least 25 percent less of that nutrient. For example, 1 tablespoon of regular mayonnaise contains 100 calories. Therefore, the reduced-calorie version must contain 75 or fewer calories.
- **"Use by" date.** This means that the product will stay fresh until that date, only if it remains unopened and stored properly. After it's been opened, you should use it quickly. Dry, packaged foods are safer to use past their "sell by" or "use by" dates. It's normally the

moisture in food that causes rapid spoilage. However, the longer you keep dry, packaged foods open, the more the quality of the food will deteriorate. (*Note of caution:* Refrigeration won't keep the food indefinitely. Bacteria still grows in cold conditions, even in the freezer.)

chapter 25

Food Focus

If your eyes hurt after you drink coffee, you have to take the spoon out of the cup.

—Norm Crosby

Certain cultures and countries in the world have a lower incidence of some of the major diseases compared to America. That raises the question as to what they're doing differently. The first thing researchers tend to look at is what those people are eating. Being able to study foods under a microscope prompts scientists to ask what particular compounds are in the foods that seem to have health-giving properties. This chapter covers some of the foods that have been in the news lately and things you might want to consider when you go to the grocery store.

Yearning for Yogurt

Yogurt, which used to be considered the food of the hippie vegetarian and food faddist, is now accepted by all generations. Its history lies in the Balkans, where it's one of the staples in the Bulgarians' diet. In the early twentieth century, the Western world was made aware of the increased life span of

Bulgarians. Was it the yogurt? We've since learned that the live bacteria culture used in making yogurt is beneficial to the bacteria in human intestines. Women have even found yogurt to be valuable in preventing vaginal yeast infections.

Isaac Carasso, who had lived in the Balkans and eaten yogurt, took the recipe with him to Barcelona in about 1919, where he introduced the Spanish to yogurt. He produced a product under the name Danone, meaning "Little Daniel," after his son. When his son, Daniel, immigrated to the United States in 1942, he started a yogurt company in the Bronx, renaming the product Dannon to make it sound more American. At that time, the yogurt was plain, tart, and sold in 8-ounce glass jars. The product didn't take off until 1947 when Dannon added fruit on the bottom. American taste buds seemed to prefer the sweeter, less-tart flavor. (It may say something about our dependency on sugar.) In 1955, a low-fat variety was introduced for the health enthusiast. What was considered their most successful launch was Dannon "Light," a low-fat version made with the artificial sweetener aspartame. Since then, efforts have been made by the company to appeal to the kids' market by adding toppings and by putting yogurt in squeezable tubes.

> Look for yogurt with the highest %DV for calcium, the lowest %DV for saturated and total fat, and the lowest amount of sugar. Skip the yogurt with goodies like candy, cookies, and sprinkles. Your best bet is to buy nonfat or low-fat plain yogurt and add your own fresh fruit. If you want crunch, sprinkle some Post Grape-Nuts cereal, low-fat granola, or sunflower seeds on top.

One of Dannon's major competitors is General Mills' Yoplait yogurt. They, too, have fat-free, low-fat, and regular varieties; yogurt-in-a-tube; yogurt drinks; yogurt with cereal; and other varieties. The yogurt market is very competitive, especially now when some studies are finding that there may be a connection with the intake of calcium and weight loss.

Water, Water Everywhere

As early as 1835, Queen Victoria, who was worried that her drinking water was unsafe, commissioned John Doulton to produce filtered water for the royal household. Doulton was a fine china maker who used his knowledge of earth and clay to create a water-filtration system. I wonder what Doulton would say if he were alive today, regarding the plethora of bottled water sold in stores. Although it encourages people to drink more water than they might normally drink, most of the water supply in the United States is quite safe. Of course, whether you like the taste of the water may be another story. I think that's why Perrier became the water of choice as we boomers were maturing, besides being quite chic!

To keep our water safe, cities must chlorinate it to kill off bacteria. Some areas even put fluoride in the water, as protection against tooth decay and bone weakening. These chemicals can, and often do, alter the flavor of the water. So you might find bottled water more palatable. If you do drink from the tap and are worried about exposure to lead and other minerals, drink water only from the cold tap (because hot water contains more of these elements). Drinking from the cold tap is especially important when you have a water softener. To make water "soft," salts are added, which means you're getting more sodium than your body needs from the hot tap.

So what are you getting when you buy bottled water?

- **Mineral water** is spring water that contains a specified amount of naturally occurring minerals.
- **Purified water** is water that's been distilled by ion-exchange or reverse osmosis.
- **Sparkling water** is spring water that's had carbon dioxide added to create the bubbles.
- **Spring water** is natural water that surfaces from underground water deposits.

As if it's not enough to have these various types of water, leave it to the food manufacturers to give us even more to choose from. Water now comes with an assortment of nutrients, herbs, flavors, and sweeteners. But best of all are the names given to these waters to make you think you'll be the healthier for drinking them. Have some "fitness water," "vitamin water," or "energy water." All this "enhancing" costs you a lot, and your body is truly no better off. You'd be best to stick with food to get your nutrients. And you certainly shouldn't be paying for water with sugar that's just going to put the weight on.

There are also home water-filtration systems that you can attach to your water system or your faucet. There are standalone containers that have a filter. You'll never get all the contaminants out, but you can remove enough to improve the taste of your water. Don't forget to change the filter and clean the container regularly to avoid bacterial growth. Otherwise, deposits will build up and the filter will no longer be functional or safe.

As to how much fluid you should drink, the recommendation from most authorities is 4 cups for every 1,000 calories of food you eat. Any fluid can make up part of that recommendation. It can be juice, milk, and other beverages. Exercise increases the amount of fluid you need. You should drink some fluid before you exercise, while you're exercising, and afterward. It's not unusual for someone who's exercising for 60 minutes to drink at least 5 cups water. And don't rely on thirst to be your guide. As you get older, your thirst barometer becomes less efficient. However, there are ways for you to know you're not getting enough water—having a low volume of urine, getting muscle cramps easily (especially in the legs), and having deeply colored urine (unless you're taking over 100% Daily Value of the B vitamins, which make your urine more yellow) are a few symptoms to watch out for.

A clever way to be sure you're drinking enough water is to put 6 to 8 cups water in a container in your refrigerator. By the end of the day, you should have drained it dry. Then you know you got enough.

Appreciate that some of the fluid your body needs will come from the foods you eat. Certain fruits and vegetables are very high in water. In fact, watermelon didn't get its name for nothing. It's about 90 percent water.

Egg Questions

Can I eat an egg a day? Although the American Heart Association changed their tune in the year 2000, telling the American public that they could have an egg a day, they never gave up their recommendation that your total cholesterol intake should be below 300 milligrams. (If you have high cholesterol, heart disease, or diabetes, you should limit your cholesterol intake to 200 milligrams.) If you consider that

1 egg has about 213 milligrams of cholesterol, that doesn't leave much room that day for other high-cholesterol foods. Cholesterol is found only in animal products—both meat and dairy. If you really want to have meat and eggs on the same day, try using egg substitutes or just eat the egg whites.

Are eggs considered the ultimate protein? It's true that the egg is considered the "perfect" protein because it has the optimal ratio of amino acids. However, if you're eating a varied diet, you should be getting enough protein in other foods to provide you with a healthy diet without relying on eggs for your protein.

Are eggs the only food I need to worry about if I have high cholesterol? Too much dietary cholesterol can lead to elevated blood cholesterol. However, the real culprit in high blood cholesterol is saturated fat. The saturated fat you eat affects blood cholesterol far more strongly than the cholesterol you eat. If you're adventurous, you might want to try such meats as emu, bison, buffalo, antelope, goat, or venison, because they're all very low in saturated fat and total fat. Their cholesterol is comparable to beef.

Cholesterol Counts

Meats/Poultry/Seafood

4 ounces

- Fish—60 to 80 mg
- Shrimp—220 mg
- Poultry—85 to 95 mg
- Beef—80 to 140 mg
- Beef liver—440 mg
- Pork—80 to 140 mg
- Clams, crabs, lobster, or scallops—75 mg

Dairy

1 tablespoon

- Butter—35 mg
- Cream—10 mg

Other

- Whipping cream—20 mg
- 1 ounce cheese—25 mg
- 1 cup milk—15 to 35 mg

Note: The ranges are due to lower and higher fat content, depending on the cut of meat. Restaurant foods and packaged foods can run far higher than the above numbers.

Does the color of the shell say something about the nutritional quality of the egg? Whether the shell is white or brown has no effect on the nutritional quality of the egg. The breed of hen that laid it determines the shell color. "Certified organic" tells you that the hens were fed organic feed with no antibiotics. "Free range" means the hens were not raised in crowded cages. By the way, never buy eggs that have been sitting out of refrigeration.

Nuts Such a Bad Idea

Can you imagine being told now that nuts are actually good for you? For so many years we were told to lay off the nuts, partly because they're high in fat. (One ounce has about 150 to 200 calories and between 13 to 22 grams fat.) However, that fat is mostly the healthier unsaturated fat. The monounsaturated fat helps to lower the bad LDL cholesterol without also lowering the good HDL cholesterol. Brazil nuts are high in selenium and quercetin, both found to be protective against cancer. Walnuts are high in omega-3 fatty acids that are protective against heart disease. Nuts are also a good source of protein. As you saw in the Food Guide Pyramid, nuts are grouped with meats and poultry. Some nuts are even high in fiber—such as almonds, hazelnuts, and pistachios; some are high in phytochemicals.

> A water chestnut is not a nut, but part of a grassy pond plant.

Try to limit your intake of nuts to a small handful. With that said, here are some ways to get some nuts in your day. Use peanut butter as a spread on your toast instead of margarine. Top your salad, cereal, or yogurt with a sprinkling of chopped nuts. As a coating, dip a piece of fish in some egg whites and then into a mixture of crushed nuts and breadcrumbs; then brown in a skillet using a teaspoon of olive oil. Nuts also work well with pasta or rice. Try them in your pancakes or muffins, as well.

Tea Time

Tea has been the beverage of choice in China for more than 5,000 years. Americans, who've been loyal to their cup of coffee, are beginning to change camps. (Don't worry, Starbucks, America will never lose its love affair with the latté!) There may be good reasons for drinking tea. Tea is loaded with polyphenols, which act as antioxidants to protect against cancer and heart disease. Green tea has more polyphenols than black tea, but if you prefer black tea, enjoy. The stronger you make the tea, the more polyphenols are released in the water. What's nice is that having a cup of tea counts toward one cup of your fluid intake for the day.

The way tea is processed determines whether it will be green or black. Green tea has less processing done to it than black tea. The leaves are steamed quickly and then packaged. Black teas require drying, crushing, and fermenting.

By the way, tea has about one third to one half the amount of caffeine found in a cup of coffee. So if you find that caffeine keeps you up at night, have a cup of herbal tea. Just appreciate that it doesn't have the health benefits of regular tea, because herbal teas are blends of roots, leaves, flowers, and herbs. However, some herbal teas have their own benefits.

What's Being Added to Your Food

If we all grew our own produce and baked our own breads and crackers, raised our own cows and chickens, and cooked our own meals, we probably would have no need for additives. However, with the number of packaged foods Americans eat today, there's no way to maintain freshness, safety, or food texture without the use of food additives. Some of the additives that are put in our foods have been shown, in studies, to cause problems in animals; but they don't pose a big enough problem for humans to prompt the FDA to ban them from the food supply. So your best bet is to limit the number of foods you eat that are processed.

Fortification is another story. Without it, we might be a nutrient-deficient country. In the case of grains, food manufacturers have to put back in some of the nutrients—in particular, the B vitamins—they took out in the refining process of the flour. Now, folate has been included due to possible neural tube defects in newborns because the mother was deficient in folate. Folate also provides some heart protection. We're even finding it necessary to fortify many foods with calcium, such as orange juice and soda, just because Americans aren't getting enough calcium in their diet. Osteoporosis (porous bones) can be a major problem for adults, especially as we get older. Most people don't appreciate that bones are living tissue. Calcium travels in and out of them, as long as the calcium is available. If the body needs calcium for some biological process, it will pull the calcium out of the bones for it. Without enough calcium in your diet, there's nothing to go back into the bones. And now you've got the potential for osteoporosis. The National Academy of Sciences recommends that those people between 31 and 50 years old get 1,000 milligrams of calcium a day. If you're between 51 and 70 years old, you need a bit more at 1,200 milligrams. It may seem like a lot, but it is doable. The following table shows you what foods could supply you with your daily calcium needs. If you don't think you can get enough from your food, it would be wise to take a supplement to make up for the shortfall.

Sources of Calcium

Food	Amount	Calcium (mgs)
Milk and yogurt	8 ounces	300
Cheese	1 ounce	200
Fortified soy milk	1 cup	180 to 200*
Tofu, prepared with calcium	1/4 cup	125
Legumes—beans	1/2 cup	40 to 60
Salmon, canned with bones	3 ounces	190
Leafy green vegetables	1/2 cup	50 to 100
Other vegetables	1/2 cup	25 to 50
Orange juice, fortified	6 ounces	200
Blackstrap molasses	1 tablespoon	170

Ranges of calcium are averages of various sources in that food category.

**Labels may say 300 mg, but calcium from soy milk is not as well absorbed as that from cow's milk.*

chapter 26

Julia Child, Move Over

You don't have to cook fancy or complicated master-pieces—just good food from fresh ingredients.
—Julia Child

I have fond childhood memories of my grandmother's cooking. She was a fantastic baker and a good cook. When she died, my dad had her recipes typed up and bound into a book for my sisters and me. We often laughed about some of the recipe ingredients, because they'd be hard to reproduce today. One recipe, for date nut bread, calls for a 28-cent package of dates. With that recipe going back to the 1940s, I wonder what size package I'd get today. (How much has 28 cents inflated to?) Nothing was exact—a glass of this (what size glass?), a sprinkling of that (how much is a sprinkle?). Whereas my grandmother baked from scratch, my mother used packaged mixes. Pillsbury supplied the rolls, Betty Crocker provided the cake mixes, and Jell-O came out with Instant Pudding. Now even we kids could make dessert.

Do you have any fond memories of the cooking that went on in your house? What foods do you remember most? It's interesting that, although women didn't want to spend too much time in the kitchen, they still wanted to feel that they were cooking for their families. Pillsbury and Betty Crocker thought they'd make life easier for homemakers by including powdered eggs in their cake mixes. However, they found out they had taken convenience one step too far. Consumers wanted to add their own eggs—making them feel that they had participated somewhat in the cooking process. Also, it seemed like it was more "homemade" or "fresh" that way.

Today, homemakers are less concerned about appearing to be making the meal "from scratch." What we've become are assemblers. A stroll down the freezer section and aisles of your supermarket tells it all. We can now get a full-course meal all prepared (and I'm not talking about TV dinners here). You can get a fully cooked roast, twice-baked potatoes, and vegetables in sauce—and all it takes on your part is opening the packages and heating. Now I'm not saying that a meal like this is low in calories or fat, but cooking seems to be becoming a lost art.

Neither my grandmother nor my mother cooked what we would consider today as *haute cuisine*. It was family-style cooking—soups, roasts, corn on the cob, corned beef, tossed salads, steamed vegetables, barbecued meat, casseroles. Most of what they cooked didn't require a recipe. It was just a matter of putting the basic ingredients in a pot, throwing in some seasonings, and letting it cook on the back burner. Most of the time the platters or bowls of food were brought to the table so we could serve ourselves family style. (Lesson 1: If you want to lose weight, never leave platters of food on the table. It's much too easy to go for seconds and thirds.)

By the time the last of the baby boomers was born, many mothers were working. So food manufacturers developed recipes to show women how they could use shortcuts to get the meal on the table quickly. Canned foods were the answer. Campbell's was a big proponent of this, pushing their soup line as a way of putting together a casserole. One popular cookbook in the 1950s was Poppy Cannon's *The Can-Opener Cookbook*. The title speaks for itself. Not long after her cookbook was published, the first electric can opener was sold to consumers.

By the 1960s, it seemed there was a renewed interest in more elegant cooking (on the weekends when more time was available). It could be that after Jackie Kennedy brought a French chef to the White House, American women wanted to imitate her in a way they could. (These women all wore the pillbox hat made so popular by Jackie. Why not the cooking style, too?) During the week, our mothers would rely heavily on mixes and frozen dinners. On the weekend, they'd experiment with more elegant foods (and finally have a use for their formal dining room). Julia Child was there in 1963, debuting her cooking show on television. She showed women how to make recipes from her cookbook, *Mastering the Art of French Cooking,* and impress their family and friends. She made cooking seem fun.

She was not alone on the TV airwaves. A man from Australia, named Graham Kerr, known to his audience as the "Galloping Gourmet," would crack jokes and drink wine while he cooked. He was the early day Emeril Lagasse. Whereas Child was on in the evening, Kerr appealed to the daytime watchers. Some of us boomers were finally old enough to start taking an interest in this thing called cooking. (Now, you can tune into the Food TV Network and watch cooking programs 24 hours a day. Some of the shows are quite entertaining, but some of the recipes they share are challenging enough that even restaurants might not try them. You have to wonder how Martha Stewart could tell us how to gold leaf our gingerbread houses or mold candy when we're lucky enough just to find the time to cook a basic meal. Oh well, call it good theater.)

Child and Kerr seemed to rekindle an interest in cooking. Even though many men had been exposed to foreign flavors (from European to Asian) during World War II, it wasn't until the 1960s that people started experimenting in the home with foreign cuisines (other than maybe serving spaghetti). Time-Life Books brought out the fantastic *Foods of the World* series that dedicated one volume to each country's cooking. With increased American affluence, more people were traveling to other countries and becoming acquainted with foreign foods. The number of cookbooks published each year continued to grow and, even today, is one of the largest categories of books sold. Women wanted then what we still look for in a cookbook today: recipes that are quick and easy but that result in food that tastes like we've spent hours in the kitchen preparing it. With so much in the news about weight and diseases, we also want our food to be healthful.

By the 1970s, we were dabbling in what would eventually be called *nouvelle cuisine,* a healthier approach to cooking. Maybe the hippies had some influence, feeling people should eat "closer to the land." Natural foods and home gardening became popular. Foreign foods were no longer foreign. Couscous and kiwi fruit were no longer "exotic." Some of the older boomers were becoming homeowners and parents. It was their turn to take over kitchen duty. If you wanted to learn how to cook, there were classes through the local YMCA or community center. My mother never formally taught me how to cook. I learned by watching her. To get the details that I never picked up, I took a Chinese cooking class and a bread-making class. The most fun, though, was the cake-decorating class. As I write this, I wonder how I found the time to make a basket cake full of chrysanthemums, roses, and pansies. I don't know how I'd do it today. That's where we boomers are now. Wanting to taste the finer flavors of home-cooking, but wondering what other part of our lives we'd have to give up for that pleasure.

Appliance manufacturers are trying to help. From blenders to mixers to food processors, a variety of appliances have made the jobs in the kitchen easier. However, many who have bought pasta makers, ice cream makers, and coffee grinders in hopes of making these foods fresh have found that their inspiration was lost after several attempts. Those items either are collecting dust in some closet or were sold at a garage sale.

Make It Last

The typical approach to cooking is to make enough for the meal you're preparing. Yet, think of the advantage of making two or three meals at one time. You're already having to do the preparation, and you're getting the pots dirty anyway. A few extra moments spent now means many more saved for the next meal. I'm a firm believer in leftovers (other than vegetables, which I don't enjoy reheated because they become overcooked). I've made many a multimeal recipe in my time—some that have been overwhelming successes, and others that the family said weren't worth making again. I normally put any extra amount I cooked in the freezer to be pulled out sometime later (up to several months) for a quick dinner. Oftentimes, the "loser" recipes would be met with great approval. Here's the surprise I learned. After several weeks or months in the freezer, the flavors had continued to work through the dish, and it somehow got better. Too late. I'd already thrown away the recipe. So the lesson is, don't underestimate freezing your leftovers.

> *The most remarkable thing about my mother is that for 30 years she served the family nothing but leftovers. The original meal has never been found.*
>
> —*Sam Levinson*

Many people prefer to put food away in the refrigerator for the next night. Because I don't particularly like having the same thing night after night, I get good use out of my freezer. Whether you refrigerate or freeze your leftovers, separate what you're having for dinner from that which you're storing. Then store it immediately, to keep it safe for the next time. Don't give food bugs a chance to grow.

That brings up the point of how to package food. There are so many ways to store food—from plastic storage bags to aluminum foil and plastic containers. Thanks to a man named Earl W. Tupper, we have Tupperware and all the knockoffs we see today. Back when the first boomers were being born, Tupper invented a lightweight and sturdy polyethylene plastic that he made into food-storage containers. Before his invention, food had to be stored in clunky, breakable glass containers. What made his product unique was his "Tupper seal" that gave the containers an airtight closure. He tried selling his products in department stores, with little success, because people didn't know how to "burp" the cover. It's when Brownie Wise, a single mother, suggested he sell the product at home parties that the product and the company took off. Do you have a Tupperware container at home? I received a number of them when I got married and they're still going strong. Unfortunately, you can now get throwaway containers—and add to the landfill. Please consider washing and reusing them, instead.

You might want to try storing soups the way I do. After we've finished drinking a half-gallon container of milk, I thoroughly wash and dry the carton. I tear open the top so it gives me a wide opening. Then I pour in the soup, close the top, staple it shut, label and date each package. Then I freeze it.

If you're freezing the food, there's a point where the food quality begins to deteriorate. The texture changes, as well as the flavor. So I find it helpful to have an ongoing list of what I put into the freezer, with the date it was cooked. Then, when I take something out, I cross it off the list. I suggest you use the FIFO method—first in, first out. Try to use the oldest-dated food first.

When I pull a meal from the freezer shortly before I'm going to need it (dinner, for example), I defrost it in the microwave. This works really well for those last-minute I-forgot-to-take-something-out dinners. Why buy packaged foods when you can have the same convenience for less money? And it's homemade—seasoned the way you like it. For those people who are too busy during the week to batch cook, do it on the weekends. Of course, if you don't enjoy cooking, then packaged foods may seem heaven-sent.

Use It Twice

A variation of making one dish last for more than one meal is using the food twice. For example, if I'm making chicken soup, there's often more chicken than I need for one meal of soup. So I pick the chicken off the bones and use it to make, for example, chicken tetrazzini the next night, and then chicken Caesar salad the following night. Sometimes I'll just bag the chicken pieces and freeze them. Then I can just defrost them in the microwave when I want to make a dish calling for cut-up chicken.

Here's another easy idea. I'll often make more pasta than I need for one dinner. I put the leftovers in the refrigerator to use for another meal. To refresh and reheat the pasta, I pour hot water over it. Maybe the first night I used the pasta to make that chicken tetrazzini dish I mentioned previously. The next night I might serve it with a marinara sauce. Here's a hint for storing pasta: Stir in a little olive oil to keep it from sticking together.

Again, when you make rice, think about making more at one time than you'll need for that one dish you're making. Because it takes so long to cook, by making extra you can eliminate that time crunch for the next rice meal. Maybe the first night you make a rice pilaf; on the next night, you might make fried rice. Because the rice will have gotten quite dry, you might need to add a little water when you reheat it. Rice freezes well, so consider bagging the extra amount you made in meal-size portions. I've seen frozen rice in the market, but you can make it much more cheaply on your own.

I like making big roasts because they go so far and you can do so much with them. The first night you can serve it hot; the second night you can have hot or cold sandwiches; and the following night you can add the meat to a stir-fry, casserole, or stew.

Cutting vegetables into small pieces exposes more surface to the air and destroys some of the nutrients. So I prefer to cut up only the amount of vegetables I'll need for a particular dish. That way they're always their freshest.

Following is a week's worth of dinner menus, based on this concept of cooking it once for twice the pleasure. See if you can spot what got cooked in a first meal and used in a second meal.

Monday

Chicken soup with rice and chunks of chicken

Tossed organic greens with walnut raspberry vinaigrette

Tuesday

Chicken tetrazzini with pasta and green peas

Grilled red peppers and eggplant (make some extra and you can use it on tomorrow night's pasta primavera)

Wednesday

Roast beef

Pasta primavera

Thursday

Fried rice with chunks of ham and shrimp

Oriental chicken salad

Friday

Roast beef sandwich au jus

Vegetable medley

Variations on a Theme

I like to find a style of cooking that's easy to do and lends itself to different seasonings. I've found that making a stir-fry, a stew, and a soup fits those requirements. They're easy approaches to cooking that require very little effort. I'll be sharing with you the basic recipe for each of these styles in a moment.

After you have the basic style of cooking down, varying the seasonings according to the different ethnic cuisines gives you the "variation on a theme." The following list should help. Consider using a combination of the seasonings suggested for the cuisine of your choice. If you can, choose fresh herbs when they're available. Whether fresh or dried, herbs have some health benefits because of their antioxidant activity.

- **Chinese.** Soy sauce (for those on low-sodium diets, buy low-sodium soy sauce), ginger, garlic, hoisin sauce, sesame oil, sesame seeds
- **French.** Shallots, leek, rosemary, thyme, tarragon, sage, white wine, fat-free cream or evaporated skim milk
- **Hungarian.** Onions, paprika, dill, caraway, plain nonfat or low-fat yogurt
- **Indian.** Curry, turmeric, coumarin, chutney
- **Italian.** Basil, oregano, parsley, sun-dried tomatoes, chopped tomatoes, garlic, onions, red wine, a sprinkling of Parmesan cheese
- **Japanese.** Soy sauce, sugar (go easy on this because these are empty calories), rice cooking wine, bonito flakes, wasabi (horseradish)
- **Mexican.** Chilies, cilantro, cumin, tomatoes, onions; and toppings such as avocado, salsa, a small amount of grated cheese, or low-fat sour cream

A note about beef or chicken stock in the following recipes: If you're on a salt-restricted diet, select a low-sodium stock.

Whether you're making a stir-fry, a stew, or a soup, have your vegetables cut up and ready—they can be fresh or frozen (but thaw them before using). You can choose a medley of vegetables or one type in particular. Use about 3/4 cup per person. Have your meat (about 4 to 5 ounces per person) cut up into about the same-size chunks as the vegetables. The meat could be chicken, turkey, beef, pork, lamb, fish, or shellfish. However, be careful that you don't overcook the fish and shellfish. It's best to put them in as the last ingredient before serving. If you want to make the dish meatless, you can use firm tofu (soybean cake) for your protein. Mix in about 3/4 to one cup per person of cooked rice, pasta, potatoes, or any other starch you like. Or have your starch on the side.

Making a stir-fry. Mix together 1 tablespoon cornstarch and 1/2 cup chicken or beef stock. Set aside. Have some water or chicken or beef stock handy.

Spray a frying pan or wok (Chinese frying pan) with some vegetable oil spray and place over medium-high to high heat. Toss in the vegetables, sauté them with a little kosher salt (if you're not on a sodium-restricted diet). Depending on your choice of vegetables (for example, broccoli and carrots), you may need to put several tablespoons of the stock in the pan to steam them slightly. Cover while they steam. When cooked to a crisp and bright color, set them aside.

Spray the frying pan again with the vegetable oil spray and sauté your meat choice with a little kosher salt until it's browned on the outside and cooked on the inside. Add several tablespoons of stock to the pan to keep the meat from sticking. If you like pepper, add some of that, too. When the meat is cooked, put the vegetables back in.

Now sprinkle on your choice of seasonings, along with the cornstarch mixture. Continue to stir-fry until the liquid has thickened slightly.

Spoon the mixture over your starch choice (rice, pasta, potato, and so on) and serve.

For example, I think I'll have my stir-fry Hungarian style, choosing zucchini (thinly sliced), onion (chopped), and mushrooms (sliced) as my vegetables and two chicken breasts (cut into chunks) as the meat. (*Note:* Cut the vegetables first and set aside. Then cut the chicken. Never cut meat and other foods on the same board or with the same knife unless you have cleaned both thoroughly with soap and water.) Heat your frying pan on medium-high. First, I sauté the zucchini until just done but still crispy and set it aside in a bowl. Next I cook the onions until limp and slightly browned and put them in the bowl with the zucchini. Last, I sauté the mushrooms and add them to the rest of the vegetables. In the same frying pan, I add some more vegetable oil spray and sauté cubes of chicken until cooked, seasoning with a little kosher salt. Turn the flame under the pan down to medium-low. To my cornstarch mixture, I add about a teaspoon of paprika and 1/4 cup low-fat sour cream. Put the cornstarch mixture in with the chicken and stir until thickened. Add the vegetables and continue stirring until the vegetables are heated through. Serve over egg noodles.

Making stew or soup. The basic difference between stew and soup is the amount of liquid. As with the stir-fry, you're going to be making a one-pot meal. Place all the vegetables, the meat, and the seasonings in a 6- to 8-quart soup pot. (If you're using a piece of meat that needs a long time to cook to tenderize it, don't add the vegetables until the meat is cooked about halfway through.) If you're making a stew, add enough chicken or beef stock to cover the ingredients only halfway up. If you're making a soup, add enough chicken or beef stock to thoroughly cover the ingredients. In either case, cook over high heat until the mixture comes to a boil. Cover the pot, turn the heat down to low, and let the dish simmer, stirring occasionally.

If you haven't added the vegetables yet because you are using a cut of meat that needs more cooking time, about halfway through the time it takes to cook the meat, add them. If you want to include potatoes, cut them into small cubes and add them at the same time as the vegetables. Continue to cook until the vegetables and meat are done.

If you don't use potatoes, and prefer to use some of the "use-it-twice" rice or pasta you cooked the other night, add it about 15 minutes before the dish is completely cooked. Depending on how much liquid was soaked up in the cooking process, you may have to add more. Season to taste with salt and/or pepper.

For those who want more recipe ideas, look in Appendix L for places to search the web to find recipes.

Low-Fat Cooking Utensils

Technology has helped us to be better and healthier cooks. For example, the **microwave** can cook food without extra fat. I'm not particularly keen on the way it cooks meat (it comes out too tough for my liking), but it's marvelous on vegetables and fish, and it certainly does a great job on defrosting and reheating foods.

Then there's the **grilling machine** that doesn't require extra fat. You get those delicious-looking grill stripes on the meat, and the fat dribbles off into a dish. You might also try cooking vegetables on the grilling machine.

When I'm making soup, I always use a **defatting cup or ladle.** If you have the time, you can always put your soup in the refrigerator and wait 24 hours for the fat to rise to the surface and congeal. Then you can remove the fat layer with a fork or spoon. However, if you want to eat your soup close to the time you cook it, the defatting cup or ladle works best. You simply pour the soup into the cup or ladle and wait a minute to let the fat float to the top. The defatting cup has a spout attached at the base, so when you pour the soup out, you're really pouring from where the soup is fat free. By the time you've poured off the entire fat-free portion, the only thing left in the cup is the fat. You can throw that away. The ladle has a push-button on the handle, so the soup comes out the bottom in a similar fashion.

Nonstick frying pans allow you to cook fat free. If you need a little "greasing," you can use a vegetable oil spray or try some chicken or beef stock.

If you want to use your own oil (especially one of the herb-flavored varieties), you can buy a **mister** that you fill and use in place of the store-bought vegetable oil sprays. You can even use a **plastic refillable pump bottle.**

If you like popcorn, use a **popcorn popper** that uses air, instead of fat, to cook the corn. Then spray the popcorn with a butter-flavored vegetable oil spray, or mist it with water and sprinkle on herbs or flavored butter-substitute flakes.

Clever Cooking Tips

The following various cooking tips will help you with everything from saving time to substitutions:

- When a recipe calls for a certain amount of fat, cut that amount back by 25 to 50 percent. Try using cooking sprays when frying or sautéing. There are now even olive oil sprays. There are also flavored oil sprays (butter, basil, and so on) that provide the flavor without much fat. Try using a little broth instead of fat. If you use a nonstick pan, you might not even need any fat at all.

- If you make your own salad dressing, instead of the usual 3-to-1 ratio of oil-to-vinegar, try 50-50 of each. If you have a favorite dressing, use it in place of the oil. Then add balsamic vinegar for a rich taste. You get the flavor you like, but with fewer calories.
- To retain the moisture in chicken during the cooking process, leave the skin on. But *do* remember to remove it before you eat the chicken. The same goes for the extra fat on meat.
- Not everything has to be made from scratch, especially when you're in a hurry. The idea is to make eating simple and convenient when you don't have the time to prepare something. Use frozen or canned vegetables if you don't have access to fresh vegetables or don't have the time to clean and cut them up. However, with markets selling cut-up vegetables in the produce department, that shouldn't be a problem. If you get a packaged meal at the market, go to the produce section and buy fresh precut salad ingredients, which can serve as the side dish to your main course. Many markets even have salad bars.
- Quick cooking methods such as stir-frying, broiling, and microwaving save time and are healthy for you.
- Baste meats and poultry with stock or a broth rather than butter or fat.
- For flavor, try adding herbs, spices, or lemon juice instead of salt.
- When using ground beef to make a sauce or casserole, brown the beef in a frying pan without any extra fat. Then drain the excess fat and liquid before incorporating the beef into the dish.
- Bake meats on a rack to allow the fats to drain away.
- Brush lean roasts with a fat-free dressing, and then rub on some herbs and spices before grilling.
- Cut lower-fat meats into thin slices and pan-broil with a little broth.

- To cut down on the amount of sugar in a recipe, increase the amount of spices for added flavor (especially cinnamon and vanilla).
- Not sure what to cook tonight? If you think along ethnic lines, each night of the week could be food from a different country. Maybe Monday nights could be Chinese, Tuesday nights could be Italian, Wednesday nights Mexican, and so on.
- Chew gum (preferably sugarless) while you're cooking—to keep the food in the pot and not in your mouth.
- After you've worked with raw meat, poultry, seafood, or eggs, wash your hands with soapy water before you do anything else with your food. There are bacteria to worry about. And don't forget to always wash your cutting board, knives, and other utensils you've used, especially before cutting raw vegetables and other foods.
- Even if you don't plan to eat the skin of fruits and vegetables, scrub them so you don't transfer any bacteria into the meaty part of the produce. This goes for melons, as well. You may be tempted to try produce cleaners. Although they may clean off dirt, fingerprints, and wax, you can accomplish the same thing by rinsing your produce really well under running water. Produce sprays don't get rid of harmful bacteria any better than a good washing.

For more great cooking-ingredient substitutions, read Chapter 18.

chapter 27

Eating on the Run

I went into a McDonald's yesterday and said, "I'd like some fries." The girl at the counter said, "Would you like some fries with that?"

—Jay Leno

All you have to do is look at the statistics to see that more and more Americans are eating away from home. According to the USDA Food Consumption Survey, "What We Eat in America," in 1994 and 1995, 57 percent of Americans ate away from home on any given day compared to 43 percent in 1977 and 1978. It may not surprise you that fast-food restaurants, including pizza parlors, are the most frequented source for food outside the home today.

The concept of eating out started to change when the first boomers were born. Before World War II, only the rich could afford to eat in fancy restaurants. After the war, with the growth of affluence, more people had the money to eat away from home. But at the same time, there was a move away from formal dining to a more casual, laid-back style of eating, both at home and out. Coffee shops and diners were popular, as were lunch counters in drugstores and five-and-dime stores. I can still remember, as a kid, sitting at the soda counter in Woolworth's and getting to watch all the activity behind the counter. It kept us amused. Customers eating at diners were also kept amused by having little jukeboxes at their table, where they could listen to the sounds of Elvis Presley, The Beach Boys, and Neil Sadaka.

Our casual style of eating then translated into "Let's eat and get on our way." We wanted our food quick, so we could move on with our lives. Actually, according to Jim Heimann in his book *Car Hops and Curb Service,* the concept of fast food had been around for a long time before we boomers were born. He said that the first "fast-food" restaurant happened by accident in a drugstore in Memphis, Tennessee, in 1905. The drugstore was doing such fantastic business that there often were no seats available at the soda counter. So the owner allowed men to take orders out to their ladies waiting in carriages. Another restaurant, The Pig Stand, in Dallas, Texas, made a business of serving pork sandwiches to people in their cars. The owner figured that people who drove cars must be naturally lazy and would prefer not having to come inside. Drive-ins got Americans used to eating in their cars, and the habit hasn't changed. Look at how many automobiles today have cup holders. In fact, I just heard recently that some car manufacturers are putting in larger cup holders to accommodate the supersize drinks.

Making History

The serve-you-in-your-car type of drive-in restaurants faded out in the 1950s. Self-service restaurants were becoming more popular, continuing to cater to our hurry-up mentality. It was really the story of McDonald's that made franchise history in the self-service restaurant business. Richard and Maurice McDonald, in San Bernardino, California, set the standard for self-service drive-ins. When Ray Kroc came to sell them a milkshake maker in 1954, he realized what a great operation they had and suggested they franchise. At first they resisted, but eventually allowed Kroc to sell the franchises. In 1961, Kroc bought the name McDonald's from the brothers and the rest, as they say, is history.

What was equally innovative was Wendy's installing drive-thru windows in 1971. What a convenience; and now people didn't have to get out of their cars to get the food.

The Start of Fast-Food Restaurants

1950: Dunkin' Donuts

1951: Jack in the Box

1952: Church's Fried Chicken and Kentucky Fried Chicken

1953: Burger King

1954: Shakey's

1955: McDonald's and Mister Donut

1958: Pizza Hut

1965: Subway

1969: Wendy's

Just an interesting aside: Shakey's pizza chain, which was the first franchised pizza restaurant, got its name from the nickname of its founder, Sherwood Johnson. He was an ex-GI who had suffered severe malaria during the war, causing tremors. From that, he got the nickname "Shakey."

As fast-food restaurants make food more affordable, they're contributing to the obesity epidemic in the United States. For just pennies more, you can supersize your meal—get more fries, a bigger soda, a dessert parfait. This is value marketing that's too easy to be sucked into. While your wallet is contracting, your waistband is expanding. Do you ever think "How can I turn down such a deal?" Then think about taking advantage of the great price by splitting the meal with someone. Remember, it's no bargain when it puts extra pounds on you. Besides, let's talk about what makes for a healthy meal. Where are the vegetables in a fast-food meal? That one thin slice of tomato and one leaf of iceberg lettuce don't count for much. And the fries you're having aren't considered a vegetable—they're a starch.

I hate to even think about the total amount of fat you're eating in just one meal. No, let's take a moment and think about the fat. If you have a Big Mac, a large order of fries, and a supersize soda, you're getting about 1,540 calories, with one third of those calories (about 60 grams) coming from fat. You figured out the number of calories you could have for the day in Chapter 16. For some of you, this one meal would be your whole day's intake. If you consider that you should distribute your calories fairly evenly throughout the day, lunch should only use up about one third of your daily allowance. What does one third amount to for you?

Now I don't want you to think that you can never go to McDonald's or any other fast-food restaurant again. But think in terms of what you could eat that would fit into your calorie requirements. Also, keep in mind that your meal should include some vegetables. So what would you choose to eat at McDonald's? My first suggestion would be to have a chicken salad to get both your protein and vegetables. However, if you really had your heart set on a sandwich and fries, then what about the Chicken McGrill, small fries, a small green salad with light balsamic vinaigrette, and a diet soda? You could trim that 1,540 calories down to 700 calories with 35 grams of fat. You could skip the sandwich spread and lower the fat by a bit. It's still high, and it means you're going to have to be mighty careful with what else you eat during the day. Ask the restaurant for their Nutrition Facts information (most fast-food restaurants have them printed on a brochure) to see what would fit into your calorie allowance. If you can't get one, refer to Appendix L to go online for the information.

Let's not forget about the fast-food restaurants that actually are offering healthier fare. You've heard about Jared, the Subway guy? He didn't lose weight on the meatball sub sandwiches, but he did find some low-fat choices at Subway that give you a generous amount of veggies along with the meat on freshly baked rolls. Several of Arby's sandwiches are reasonably low fat, such as their grilled chicken and roast turkey sandwiches. I'm sure you can find restaurants in your area that offer healthy selections, but it's up to you to choose them.

If you're having pizza, there are ways to make it a bit lower in fat. Instead of having it with a cheese-filled crust, extra cheese, meatballs, pepperoni, or sausage, consider having some of these toppings:

artichoke hearts, Canadian bacon, grilled chicken, mushrooms, onions, pineapple, or sliced tomatoes.

The oldest of us baby boomers can no longer say that our kids are dragging us to the fast-food restaurants. Most of our children are grown and on their own. Maybe the youngest of the baby boomers still have children at home and have that pressure. With chauffeuring kids to ball practice, games, or music lessons, grabbing food on the run has become part of the routine. It seems to be true even for those without kids. I would love to see you plan your day in advance, preparing and packing a meal if you could. Make your own sandwiches, so you can control what goes in. Buy precut vegetables in the market. Add a piece of fruit. Can you make a meal out of something from last night's leftovers? In fact, next time you make dinner, make extra for lunch the next day. Think of the time and money you'll save versus waiting in the drive-thru lane, as well as the fact that you're eating healthier.

If you don't have time for that, then choose wisely at a fast-food restaurant and think about sitting down at a table. It's better than skipping lunch or dinner and opting for food from a vending machine that has little redeeming nutritional value. Set a good example for your kids. What you do is what they'll do—they're watching. You're trying to lose weight. I'm sure you don't want to see them in the same boat. Besides, do you really enjoy dashboard dining, balancing a burger with one hand and steering the car with the other, while possibly clutching a cell phone to your ear? Let's not forget that while food is for nourishment, it would be nice if you also received some pleasure from it.

> Did your family sit down to eat dinner together when you were young? Or were the scenes of dinnertime in such television shows as *Father Knows Best* or *Leave It to Beaver* pure Hollywood? Is it that today's family is less concerned about good nutrition, because they care more about other aspects of their lives? As a nutritionist, I fear the outcome. To steal a couple words from a famous bear, "Only you can prevent … health problems."

You Don't Have to Sneak Your Snacks

Snacking can be a healthy part of your diet. In fact, I recommend it if you're hungry between meals. (But a word of caution: A study was done in France that showed that if you eat a snack when you're *not* hungry, you might eat just as much at the next meal as you would have without eating a snack. And the calories from the snack you ate will just be put away into storage.) As I mentioned earlier in the book, maintaining a consistent blood sugar level is a much healthier way to go than eating too much at one meal, getting a spike in blood sugar, only to have it drop precipitously and cause you to be ravenous by the next meal. This can potentially set you up to eat too much at that meal. Of course, the calories you eat as a snack count toward your total calorie allowance for the day.

So how are you going to make the snack choice? First, I think it depends on what you have in mind. Are you looking for something sweet or salty? Bland or spicy? Chewy or crunchy? Cold or hot? My feeling is that to eat just anything, and come away dissatisfied, makes those calories a waste. (There's no reason you can't find something that's both pleasurable and nutritious.) You also run the risk of eating something else because you weren't satisfied with the first thing you ate. Create a table for snack ideas that will be handy when you get a "snack attack." Make the table five columns wide and five rows high. Label the columns "Salty," "Sweet," "Tart or Sour," "Bland," and "Fruity." Label the rows "Crunchy or Crispy," "Chewy," "Liquid or Juicy," "Creamy or Smooth," and "Soft or Melts in Your Mouth." Now fill in the table with your ideas.

Most people think that snacks have to be salty or sweet. However, there are other foods that make for great snacks that come in bite-size packages naturally, such as baby carrots, cherry tomatoes, string beans, or fruit. Then there is string cheese or crackers. In fact, almost any food will work as a snack as long as you remember what a snack is meant to be—something that will tide you over until the next meal. In other words, a snack is *not* a meal. No matter what the advertisement says about "Betcha can't eat just one," be careful how much you do eat. (Do you know what food advertisement had that slogan? Check for the answer at the end of this chapter to see if you're right.)

This is when label reading is going to be really important. When you're standing in the grocery store trying to decide between, say, Fritos

Corn Chips or Baked Lay's, check out the calories and grams of fat. They're both salty and crunchy, if that's the flavor and texture you want. However, the baked potato chips won't set you back in calories and fat as much as the corn chips. If you opt for pretzels, you might do even better. If you have to have a dip, go for the salsa or try mixing low-fat yogurt instead of sour cream with your dip mix.

Potato chips have been around much longer than most of us realize. George Crum, a chef at the elegant resort Moon Lake Lodge in Saratoga Springs, New York, invented the original potato chip in 1853. A guest kept asking Crum to make his thick French fries thinner and thinner. Out of frustration, Crum decided to make them laughably thin. Yet, the guest and others fell in love with them. It became a specialty of the house. With the invention of the mechanical potato peeler in the 1920s, potato chips could be made in bulk. For many years, potato chips remained pretty much a New England specialty until Herman Lay, a traveling salesman, tasted them and fell in love with the product. He peddled them out of the trunk of his car to grocers in the South, until his business became too big. In 1961, he merged with Frito to become Frito-Lay Inc.

Watch out for snack foods that sound healthy but aren't. For example, some fruit chips aren't simply dried fruit—they're *fried* fruit. Avoid snacks that are high in saturated fat. Don't forget about portion sizes. It's best if you count out the number of chips you should have; then put the bag away before you start eating. Otherwise, before you realize it, your hand will be scraping the bottom of the bag.

By the way, don't treat a snack as a grab-and-go food. It deserves just as much attention as your meal. Whenever you eat, take the time to notice what you're eating, and be sitting down while you do it. And I don't mean sitting at your desk working or when you're reading or watching television. The idea is that whenever food goes in your mouth, that's all you're doing. Make food an important part of your day—not a "side dish." How many times have you wandered past the refrigerator, opened the door to see what was there, and just started nibbling directly from the refrigerator on foods you found? (Sometimes you're not even hungry.) Just remember, calories count whether you're sitting down, standing up, or walking about.

Protein bars have become big business. But they weren't the first bars on the market. Granola bars probably started off the rage. Cereal bars (such as Kellogg's Nutri-Grain Bars) followed that. Close on its heels were diet bars (for example, Slim-Fast), and then came energy bars (like Power Bars). What's unfortunate is that they all seem to be headed toward being reincarnated candy bars. As we boomers are getting older, we're tending to pay a little more attention to what we eat. Just sitting down to a candy bar seems too unhealthy. However, when it masquerades as a health bar or energy bar, it seems a more justifiable snack. With the candy coating on many of these bars, the calories and saturated fat can be as high as a candy bar.

Healthy Trail Mix

1 cup pretzel sticks

1/2 cup nuts (try soy nuts for variety)

1/4 cup raisins

1/4 cup dried pineapple

1/4 cup dried cherries

2 cups Cheerios

To be fair, granola bars aren't as bad as a candy bar when it comes to the saturated fat content. Yet leave it to the food manufacturers to ruin it by adding chocolate chips and brand-name candies, such as M&Ms, to the mix. Cereal bars, in most cases, are glorified fruit Pop-Tarts. With a little bit of cereal mixed in with flour wrapped around a jamlike filling, people are fooling themselves when they think they're having a healthy breakfast. Granted, at least they're not candy coated. As a snack, maybe they're okay, if you select brands that are low in calories. Likewise, if you're going to eat a diet, protein, or energy bar for a snack, keep in mind that they're very high in calories. And as a meal replacement, they have a lot that's goes against them. They're often high in saturated fat and, I ask you again, "Where are the vegetables?"

Think Slow

If I were watching a movie of the many years that have passed since we boomers were born, I get the sense that, in our more recent years, the projector has been switched to high speed. When we were younger, it seemed that life moved at a more leisurely pace. Now, it seems we can't stuff enough in a day to satisfy us. We put ourselves under tremendous pressure to do it all. Yet we can't, and something is sacrificed. I think the way we eat and the respect for nutrition have been the biggest losers in this rat race we call life. I'm not just talking about the food we choose, but the way we enjoy it.

There is actually an international movement called Slow Food that was started in 1986 by the Italians. They were in an uproar when McDonald's wanted to locate their golden arches right next to the historic Spanish Steps in Rome. To the Italians, this was an intrusion on their cuisine and culinary history. Europeans, generally, dine—they don't inhale their food as Americans tend to do.

The movement has grown to more than 650,000 members in 45 countries, with 65 chapters in the United States. Although some believe the movement started as a humorous protest to the spread of fast food throughout the world, its objective is to save the world's unique food products that take time and artisanship to make. It's a movement to make people appreciate their local foods and traditions. Farmers' markets are just one way that allows people to share the fruit of the land in its natural state. Maybe if more people experienced unprocessed foods they'd be less accepting of what they find on many shelves in the grocery store. But it takes a different mind-set to appreciate good food. You have to slow down to really taste your food. And if you slow down, you just might find more pleasure in the company of your family and friends. You also might eat less.

Ways to Have a Slow-Food Attitude

- Always sit down at a table to eat.
- Learn to cook, so you can control what you're eating.
- Savor the flavors of what you're eating. Don't rush your meal.
- Frequent your farmers' markets and experience the local foods.
- Consider the health benefits of the foods you eat.

Answer: Frito-Lay Lays Potato Chips

chapter 28

Dining Out Means Sitting Down to Eat

Nouvelle Cuisine, roughly translated, means: I can't believe I paid ninety-six dollars and I'm still hungry.

—Mike Kalin

The United States is a great place to live. Being such a melting pot of ethnicities, we have lots of food choices when we eat out. Unfortunately, many of the ethnic restaurants have Americanized the "old country" recipes. The result is that we end up with foods that aren't nearly as healthy as the original. Many studies have shown how people from other countries who come to live in the United States lose the health advantage of their culture and experience more of the typical American health risks. And eating out a lot means it's too easy to rack up calories, eat less healthfully, and gain weight.

Dine with a Plan

Before discussing the different ethnic cuisines, let me share with you some methods of preparation or descriptions that you might find on a menu. The idea is to make you stop and question whether you're about to make the healthiest choice.

Avoid These Methods of Preparation	
Alfredo sauce	In drawn butter
Au gratin	In pastry crust
Battered and fried	Made with butter
Béchamel sauce	Made with coconut milk
Breaded and fried	Mayonnaise sauce
Butter sauce	Newburg
Buttered	Pan-fried
Buttery	Phyllo dough
Casserole	Pot pie
Cheese sauce	Prime
Cream sauce	Sizzling
Crème fraiche	Stuffed
Crispy	Stuffed and fried
Deep-fried	Stuffed with cheese
Escalloped	Tempura style
Fried to a golden crust	Thermidor
Fritters	Topped with shredded cheese
Guacamole sauce	With bacon or sausage
Hash	With sour cream
Hollandaise sauce	Wrapped in pastry dough

Try These Methods of Preparation Instead	
Au jus	In its own juices
Baked	Kabobs or skewered
Barbecued	Marinara sauce
Blackened	Marinated
Boiled	Poached
Braised	Roasted
Broiled	Sautéed

Try These Methods of Preparation Instead	
Cajun style	Served with salsa
Charbroiled	Simmered
En brochette	Smoked
Fish sauce	Steamed
Grilled	Stir-fried (ask chef to go easy on the oil)
Hot sauce	Vegetarian style
In clear broth	With herbs

An important thing to remember when you dine out—you're paying the bill and should have the meal prepared your way. The reason for eating out is so you don't have to cook the meal yourself or do the cleaning up. But that doesn't mean that you shouldn't have a say in how the food is prepared. Fortunately, most restaurants will try to accommodate your requests. So don't be afraid to ask how a dish is prepared and whether some changes can be made that will make the dish lower in fat and calories. Use some of the terms I just listed to help you out.

Ask for dressings, sauces, and toppings served on the side. Dip your fork into the dressing or sauce before you pick up the food. You'll end up eating much less of the dressing or sauce, but you'll still get the flavor.

Just because you're eating out doesn't mean you can throw all caution to the wind and overdo it. If you're eating out several times a week, then restaurant dining shouldn't be treated as a "special occasion," allowing no-holds-barred eating. And eliminate from your thinking the idea that "because I'm paying for this, I'm going to get my money's worth," and then proceed to eat until you're stuffed. Don't forget what I shared about portion control in Chapter 17: Ask for a doggie bag before you start eating. If you're afraid of overeating when you dine out, eat a light snack (think of it as an hors d'oeuvre) before you leave home.

I have often found that as I read the menu, none of the entrées are grabbing my attention and saying "I'm what you want." However, the appetizers sound so much more appealing. There's absolutely no reason why you can't make a meal of appetizers. Because appetizers are designed to be smaller than the entrées, you won't be overeating ordering this way. You might consider calling the restaurant ahead of time to have them fax you a copy of their menu. You can study the menu and have some idea what you're going to order before you get there. On-the-spot ordering (when the restaurant smells so good) might get you into trouble.

Try this the next time you go out to eat. Order only one course at a time. After you've had a salad, for example, judge how much more you need to eat to satisfy any remaining hunger. And do be honest. Don't think, "But all I've had is the salad course. My meal is not complete." Look at the menu again and order according to your real hunger level, not your eyesight appetite. The problem is that when you enter a restaurant, you're probably very hungry, and you're more likely to order too much all at once. Everything sounds good. If you really want dessert, split it with someone at the table. But remember, don't order dessert until you've finished with your meal and can judge whether you really and truly have room. If you need something sweet to finish with, try an after-dinner mint or order some fruit.

Your choice of where you eat may also influence how healthfully you eat, so make the choice wisely. You may want to avoid the all-you-can eat restaurants or buffets that allow your "eyes to be bigger than your stomach."

The remainder of the chapter shares with you how to eat more healthfully from the different cuisines of the world. Because there are so many different foods one could get at a restaurant, I can only share a handful. My focus is on providing you with ideas on what alternatives you could select to replace the higher-fat or higher-calorie choices. Therefore, you won't see listed all the healthy options. That would be a book all by itself. Just use your judgment and ask your server if you're not sure.

American Cuisine

Considering that the United States is such a melting pot, it's somewhat hard to say what foods are truly American. We can lay claim to foods such as hamburgers, fried chicken, steak, and corn-on-the-cob. And Americans can pretty much take credit for the rise of fast-food restaurants.

Different regions of the United States often showcase their local produce, seafood, and meats, but serve them in ways characteristic of their area. For example, even though both Northwest and Southwest cuisines emphasize fresh ingredients, each area handles those ingredients in unique ways. Northwest cuisine uses fresh herbs, whereas Southwest cuisine tends to be spicier. In some cases, the flavors come from a fusion of a number of cuisines. So the following list of American cuisine is fairly short. Best to look under the appropriate ethnic cuisine for more information. For example, nachos or fried mozzarella sticks may be served at an American-style restaurant, but are truly of Mexican or Italian origin.

	Instead of This ...	Try This
Breads	Basket of bread	Limit your intake to one roll or one slice of bread. If necessary, ask the waitperson to take the bread from the table to remove temptation (that is, if everyone else at the table is agreeable). *And* Ask for margarine instead of butter, to lower your intake of saturated fat.
	Hush puppies or biscuits	Whole-wheat roll
Salads	Cobb salad	Ask that it be served without the bacon and cheese and that these be replaced with more tomatoes and sprouts; have the dressing served on the side.
	Cole slaw Potato salad Tuna salad	Tossed green salad with dressing on the side
Entrées	Beef spareribs	Baby back pork spareribs (Although still high in fat, they're less than beef ribs.)
	Crab cakes	Steamed crab with cocktail sauce
	Fried chicken	Grilled chicken
	Fried shrimp	Shrimp jambalaya *Or* Steamed shrimp with cocktail sauce

	Instead of This …	Try This
Entrées	Porterhouse or T-bone steak	Filet mignon or tenderloin (Cut serving in half and immediately put half in your doggie bag. Restaurants always serve far too much meat in a serving.) *Or* Veal steak (if available, though it is pricey)
Sandwiches	Cheeseburger	Plain hamburger without dressing, but plenty of lettuce and tomatoes *Or* Grilled chicken sandwich, without mayonnaise, but with plenty of lettuce, tomatoes, and sprouts
	Sandwiches	Request whole-wheat bread, add tomatoes and sprouts, AND Leave off the mayonnaise.
		Avoid tuna salad and chicken salad, because of all the mayonnaise; better to have roast beef, ham, or turkey, without any cheese.
Vegetables	Corn-on-the-cob dripping with butter	Ask for corn-on-the-cob steamed, with no butter
	French fries (Even though Americans have taken on french fries as their own, they were originally a Belgian creation, served with mayonnaise.)	Baked potato served with margarine instead of butter (Ask for the margarine to be served on the side.)
Desserts	Cheesecake	Fruit pie (Avoid all, or at least some, of the crust.)
	Hot-fudge sundae	Sorbet

Chinese Cuisine

If Americans actually ate traditional Chinese food in China, they would be amazed at how much less fat and soy sauce are used than in the Chinese food prepared in our restaurants. Fortunately, no matter where you eat Chinese food, the focus is not on the protein part of the dish, but on the vegetables and such carbohydrates as noodles or rice. And even if a dish is high in fat, the saturated fat tends to be quite low. With the typical large serving size in American restaurants, portion control may be challenging, unless you have enough diners at the table. Of course, if you suffer from "I'm going to be sure to get my fair share on the first go-around (just in case there won't be enough for a second chance)," the likelihood is you'll end up eating far too much.

Think variety rather than quantity. Try sampling one of this and one of that. Go sparingly on the deep-fried items, and realize that many of the chicken dishes are made from the higher-fat thigh and leg portions. Tofu is a good vegetable source of protein, and it isn't high in saturated fat. Look for vegetable dishes on the menu. Ask for take-out cartons (Chinese doggie bags). That way you'll eat less and get another meal out of this one.

Even though stir-frying is healthier than deep-frying, many Chinese restaurants use a great deal of oil in the process. (Fortunately, they use mostly peanut oil, high in monounsaturated fat, which is thought to help lower blood cholesterol.) Ask whether less can be used. Noodle dishes are like sponges when oil is around. If a dish is made by coating the meat with flour or cornstarch and then fried (such as in sweet and sour pork), ask whether the dish can be stir-fried. Many dishes are made with sweet sauces, which increase the number of calories. Scrape off some of the sauce, if possible, so you can still enjoy the flavor without all the calories.

The high level of sodium in Chinese food can be a problem for individuals on severely restricted-sodium diets. It's best to limit your consumption of soup, a very high source of salt. Because most of the sauces are made with soy sauce, you can't avoid sodium entirely. You might want to avoid dishes made with bean sauce, hoisin sauce, or oyster sauce. With Chinese food being pretty much cooked to order, ask your waitperson whether less sauce can be used and whether MSG can be left out.

	Instead of This …	Try This
Appetizers	Sizzling rice soup (It sizzles because the rice has been deep-fried.)	Wonton soup
	Egg rolls (spring rolls)	Egg foo yung (Ask them to go easy on the oil.)
	Fried wontons	Potstickers (stuffed noodle packets that are browned and steamed) *Or* Steamed dumplings
Entrées	Chinese chicken salad	Ask that the deep-fried rice sticks that top the salad be served on the side.
	Deep-fried tofu and vegetables	Steamed tofu and vegetables
	Fried noodles	Steamed noodles, lo mein noodles, or vegetable chow mein
	Fried rice with ham and shrimp *Or* Fried rice with vegetables	Steamed rice
	Cashew chicken	Ask for the nuts to be served on the side and try to limit the quantity to 1 tablespoon.
	Dishes made with duck	Ask whether chicken can be substituted.
	General Tsao's chicken (cubes of chicken coated with flour, deep-fried, and served in a spicy sauce)	Szechuan chicken (cubes of chicken, stir-fried and served in a spicy sauce); go easy on the cashews.
	Kung pao (prawns with peanuts)	Ask that the peanuts be served on the side, so you can decide how much to add *Or*

	Instead of This ...	Try This
		Shrimp in garlic sauce
	Orange crispy beef	Broccoli beef
	Peking duck served with wrappers	Moo shu pork served with wrappers
	Sweet and sour pork	Barbecue pork slices
Cooking	Anything made with monosodium glutamate (MSG) and large quantities of soy sauce	Ask for dishes to be made without MSG and less soy sauce.

French Cuisine

Classic French cuisine is considered *haute cuisine,* literally "high-class cooking," with its rich sauces of butter and cream, fine ingredients, and elegant presentation. A typical dinner could include many courses, with the emphasis on sauces—béarnaise, béchamel, and Mornay being among the most familiar. Originally, only wealthier French people were afforded the opportunity to indulge in such fine fare. However, the French Revolution put many chefs out of work, and soon this style of dining was introduced to the masses.

More recently, because of the time involved in cooking haute cuisine (and probably the great amount of calories), *nouvelle cuisine* was developed. It's a lighter and healthier style of French cooking. Instead of using a cream-base, sauces are reductions and the emphasis is on fresh ingredients. Presentation has become even more important. The chef is now as much an artist as a good cook, arranging bite-sized pieces of food in ways that are appealing to the eye. In the United States, you can find French cooking on most menus of continental restaurants. Because of its elegant presentation, we tend to linger longer over a meal. This allows one to actually savor the flavor, rather than follow the usual gulp-and-dash approach of fast-food restaurants. Eating more slowly may help you to eat less, as long as you listen to your body-talk, as discussed in Chapter 19.

With French cuisine, the foods in the Try This column may be a better pick than your Instead of This … selections, but appreciate that they still may not be low-fat or low-calorie.

	Instead of This …	Try This
Breads	Baguette (French bread) served with butter	Baguette without butter (Limit the number of pieces you eat.)
Soups	French onion soup with Gruyère cheese	Have without cheese or at least remove some of it. This soup is very high in sodium. *Or* Jellied consommé (jelled clear broth)
	Lobster bisque	Bouillabaisse
Appetizers	Baked brie in pastry crust	Avoid, or have a very small piece and share with others at the table.
	Escargots (snails)	Drain butter from escargots before eating.
	Paté de foie gras on toast	If you're curious about its taste, divide portion among everyone at the table, so all you eat is a sample.
Salads	Crudités (fresh vegetables served with a mayonnaise dip)	Crudités without the dip or limit yourself to 1 tablespoon
	La salade d'endive au noix	Ask for the dressing on the side.
	Salade Nicoise (salad of tuna, green beans, potato, olives, tomato)	Ask for the dressing on the side.
Entrées	Beef Wellington (fillet of beef cloaked in goose liver paté and wrapped in puff pastry)	Filet mignon topped with mushroom sauce *Or* Chateaubriand (beef) (usually served for two) *Or* Escalope de veau (veal), avoiding as much of the sauce as possible *Or* Rack of lamb in herbed breading

	Instead of This ...	Try This
Entrées	Duck l'Orange	Coq au vin (chicken in wine sauce)
	Les Coquille St. Jacques (scallops in a cream sauce)	Terrine of fruit de mer (with clams, mussels, shrimp, scallops, calamari in a lobster broth with potatoes, fennel, and carrots)
	Quiche Lorraine	Eat a very small piece
Desserts	Crème brulée (custard)	Grand Marnier soufflé
	Éclairs	Crepes Suzette (try to drain off syrupy sauce)

Italian Cuisine

If you were to travel to Italy, you'd find cuisine that reflects the specific region of Italy you were visiting. Northern Italian food traditionally is more delicate, with dishes made in butter and wine sauces or cream-based sauces. The southern part of Italy has more of the tomato-based sauces (marinara and cacciatore) and a heavier use of olive oil, oregano, basil, and garlic. Fish tends to be the major source of protein.

Our American version of Italian dining depends upon the restaurant. Less-expensive restaurants tend to cook the southern Italian style, with a heavy use of garlic. If they do provide dishes in cream sauce, the sauce is much heavier than you'd find in northern Italy. One really good example is fettuccine Alfredo. We Americans don't have a clue what that dish really is. Most restaurants here drown the noodles in a cream sauce. However, the original version, served at the original Alfredo's restaurant in Rome, is simply fettuccine tossed with butter and several types of cheeses. It's so light it nearly floats off your plate. Fortunately, upscale Italian restaurants in the United States try to imitate their origins with haute cuisine treatment.

We don't even eat the meal in the same order as native Italians. We're programmed to having our salad before dinner; but Italians begin their meal with an antipasto, followed by soup, the entrée, and then have the salad at the end as a way to cleanse the mouth. Dessert is simply cheese and fruit and/or an espresso.

The menu from an elegant Italian restaurant in the United States will often be divided into sections titled Primo, Secondo, Pasta, and so forth. Primo dishes are the appetizers, and Secondo dishes are the entrée part of the meal. If you order from the Pasta section, you'll find that the plates are normally smaller, because it's thought that this will accompany your entrée. Ask to be sure. Consider making the pasta your actual meal, with a salad or antipasto from the Primo section of the menu.

Instead of This ...		**Try This**
Breads	Bread with butter *Or* Cheesy Garlic Bread	Bread with olive oil and a splash of balsamic vinegar (Measure out 1 teaspoon oil on your plate. Make it last. That's about 10% of your daily fat allowance, and you'll certainly be having more fat with your meal.)
Appetizers	Appetizer of deep-fried mozzarella sticks	Antipasto of marinated vegetables (Avoid the salami or prosciutto if you're on a low-sodium diet.) *Or* Shellfish (clams or mussels) in a garlic wine broth *Or* Minestrone soup
Salads	Caesar salad	Caesar salad with the dressing served on the side *Or* Marinated and grilled vegetables *Or* Green salad with oil-and-vinegar dressing on the side
Entrées	Deep-fried calamari (squid)	Ask that the squid be sautéed rather than fried. *Or* Shrimp scampi (Avoid as much of the butter sauce as possible.)

	Instead of This ...	**Try This**
Entrées	Eggplant Parmesan	Steamed vegetables
	Garlic roasted chicken	Remove skin before eating.
	Anything in a cream sauce	Ask for a light wine sauce.
	Pasta with cream sauce *Or* Fettuccine Alfredo	Pasta with red sauce *Or* Ask for a dish of plain pasta; then lightly sprinkle it with Parmesan cheese and maybe add a squeeze of lemon. *Or* Fettuccine Primavera *Or* Risotto without butter and cheese *Or* Linguini with clams
	Ravioli *Or* Stuffed Cannelloni *Or* Manicotti *Or* Lasagna	Capellini (angel-hair pasta), fettuccine, spaghetti, linguine, fusilli—in a light sauce
	Spaghetti with garlic oil	Spaghetti with marina sauce *Or* Spaghetti with sun-dried tomatoes
	Veal Parmigiana	Veal Cacciatore *Or* Veal Marsala *Or* Veal Piccata
Desserts	Tiramisu	Italian ices or sorbets

Japanese Cuisine

Japanese food is probably one of the healthiest of the ethnic cuisines. It's light, delicate, not heavily seasoned, and has very little fat. Rice and vegetables form the foundation of the diet, with seafood and tofu being their main sources of protein. Beef and pork are rarely eaten, because Japan is a small island nation, which has little land to be spared for raising cattle and pigs. A wide variety of seaweeds are used in Japanese cooking, from nori (used to roll sushi) to kombu (for making dashi, a soup stock). It's interesting to see the influence that other cultures have had on Japanese cuisine. The Chinese introduced the Japanese to soy products, rice, and tea. It's said that tempura has its roots in Portuguese cuisine; however, the Japanese have created a much lighter batter.

One very important element of Japanese cuisine is its presentation—helping to set the mood of the meal. Each food is given separate attention by the dish it's served in. Various-size plates and bowls are used, including the divided "bento boxes" (probably the inspiration for our divided picnic plates). The emphasis is on variety, with small portion sizes. There's a desire to produce a calm and peaceful atmosphere for dining. Therefore, meals aren't rushed, and you just may eat less.

Even though most Japanese foods are low in fat, they may contain high amounts of salt and sugar. For example, sushi rice has sugar added to it, as does teriyaki sauce and donburi (a mixture of egg and meat that's served over rice). You might also end up with a significant amount of carbohydrates in your meal, from the rice and noodles, so consider quantity while you're eating. Because there are more healthy choices than not-so-healthy choices in Japanese cuisine, you'll find fewer foods in this table than some of the other cuisines. I've just listed those foods that you might want to consider other choices for because they may be high in fat or calories.

	Instead of This …	**Try This**
Salads	Tossed green salad with miso and mayonnaise dressing	Have the dressing on the side. Sunomono—cucumber salad with dressing of sweetened rice vinegar *Or* Pickled vegetables

	Instead of This ...	Try This
Soups	Tempura-udon (wide noodles in broth, with tempura)	Yaki-udon (wide noodles in broth, with vegetables) *Or* Miso soup (soy bean-paste soup, with bits of tofu and scallions or green onions) *Or* Yosenabe (noodles, seafood, and vegetables simmered in a broth)
Entrées	Katsu Donburi (breaded and deep-fried pork cutlet, onion, and egg, made with slightly sweet sauce, served over a bowl of white rice)	Oyako donburi (sautéed chicken, onions, and egg, made with slightly sweet sauce, served over a bowl of white rice)
	Tempura (battered and deep-fried fish and vegetables)	Sashimi (fillet of fresh fish served with wasabi—a horseradish mixture—and soy sauce) *Or* Unagi (broiled freshwater eel) Try it, it's delicious.
	Tonkatsu (breaded and deep-fried pork cutlet)	Shabu-shabu (A one-pot meal you cook at the table; ingredients include thinly sliced beef, vegetables and noodles that are cooked in a broth and then dipped in various sauces.) *Or* Sukiyaki (a one-pot meal, made with beef or chicken, vegetables and noodles in broth that's seasoned with soy sauce) *Or* Teppanyaki (meat, seafood, and vegetables cooked at your table on a griddle and served with dipping sauces) *Or* Yakitori (skewered chicken pieces, broiled or grilled with teriyaki sauce)
Desserts	Green tea ice cream	Mandarin oranges

Mexican Cuisine

With a little work, a Mexican meal has the potential of being healthy and low in fat. To make it so, you'll have to sidetrack the nachos, fried taco shells, cheese, and sour cream. Instead, focus on soft tacos filled with refried beans, shredded chicken, lettuce, and tomatoes, and topped with salsa. The staples of the authentic Mexican diet tend to be corn, beans (a great source of fiber), tomatoes, and chili peppers.

When the Spaniards arrived in Mexico, they influenced the direction Mexican cooking would take. Garlic, cinnamon, onions, and rice were integrated into Mexican cuisine. Protein doesn't dominate the plate, as is typical of North American cuisine, but fat can be of concern. Many Mexican foods are fried or use lard. Finding out from your waitperson what kind of fat is used in a particular dish may help you avoid the highly saturated fats.

The first thing to contend with at a Mexican restaurant is the basket of chips served with salsa. Before you know it, you've devoured them and the waitperson is happily replacing the empty basket with a full one. Decide, in advance, how many chips you should eat (four? six? eight?), count them out on your plate, and then have the basket removed. If there are others at the table who aren't too agreeable with that idea, then when you finish what's on your plate, that's it.

	Instead of This …	Try This
Breads	Flour tortillas (often made with lard)	Corn tortillas
	Fried tortillas	Baked tortillas, either corn or flour
	Nachos, served with melted cheese	Tostada chips with salsa
Salads	Taco salad, served in crisp tortilla shell	Taco salad (Avoid the shell; ask for it to be served without sour cream and guacamole, or limit yourself to a total of 1 tablespoon of any topping; go easy on the avocado.)

	Instead of This ...	Try This
Entrées	Chimichanga (flour tortilla filled with shredded chicken or ground beef, fried and topped with melted cheese) *Or* Tacos (fried flour tortilla filled with shredded chicken or ground beef; topped with plenty of sauce, cheese, and sour cream) *Or* Tostada (fried corn tortilla covered with meat mixture and beans and topped with lettuce and onions)	Burrito (large flour tortilla filled with refried beans and meat; topped with tomato sauce and cheese) Ask that the cheese be omitted. *Or* Enchilada (corn tortilla filled with ground beef or shredded chicken and topped with tomato sauce, cheese, and sour cream) Ask that it be served without the cheese and sour cream.
	Fajitas (flour tortilla wrapped around marinated beef or chicken with vegetables), topped with sour cream and guacamole	Fajita (Ask for it to be served without sour cream and guacamole, or limit yourself to a total of 1 tablespoon of any topping.)
Side Dishes	Refried beans	Black beans *Or* Mexican rice
	Toppings: guacamole, sour cream, shredded cheese	Salsa, chopped tomatoes, shredded lettuce Have high-fat toppings served on the side; dip your fork into the topping first, and then spear the food.
Desserts	Sopaipilla (deep-fried dough sprinkled with cinnamon and sugar)	Flan (egg custard drizzled with caramel syrup)

part 5

The Icing on the Cake

Do you realize how much you've learned so far in this book? There's just a little more I'd like you to know in order to make your weight-loss program successful. I call it the "icing on the cake," because just as icing finishes off a cake and makes it complete, this last section should do the same for you. Even though I'm a dietitian and feel nutrition is an integral part of our being, I'd be remiss if I didn't emphasize the need for exercise. I look at exercise and nutrition as a pair of shoes. Have you ever walked out the front door with only one shoe on? I doubt it. So you shouldn't think that you can lose weight by only changing what you eat. That's especially true when studies have shown that greater weight loss occurs with exercise, and the loss is better maintained with regular exercise.

How you handle stress is every bit as important as exercise in the weight-loss process. I believe there's a mind-body connection, and that to have a healthy body, you must deal with stress in a healthy manner. So I've dedicated a chapter to dealing with stress. There's also a chapter on clever diet tips, which are short sound bites you can easily incorporate into your daily routine.

chapter 29

Move It to Lose It

I had to give up jogging for my health. My thighs kept rubbing together and setting my pantyhose on fire.
—Roseanne

Have you ever thought about the strength of the jaw muscle? It's probably one of the strongest muscles in our body. When we consider how often we exercise it, it's not surprising. Think about the resistance against which we ask it to perform—from hard carrots to tough meat to chewy caramels. If we used all the other muscles in our body as consistently, we'd be in great shape.

The problem for many people is getting started. When you haven't been an exerciser, it takes a lot of mental strength to counteract the inertia of not exercising. It's hard to imagine how it will feel to be physically fit. People are very good at making excuses. Do any of these sound familiar?

Excuse: I'm too tired.

Fact: Exercise gives you energy. The more fit you are, the more you'll find you can get done.

Excuse: I don't have the time.

Fact: Every day contains 24 hours. You have the choice of what you can do with those hours. Why are you willing to spend time bathing, combing your hair, shaving, or putting on make-up—in other words, fixing the way you look on the outside—but you're not willing to spend time fixing up what's on the inside? Just consider how you prioritize the things you do, and make exercise one of those daily priorities.

Excuse: It takes too much time.

Fact: Research has shown that you can accumulate physical activity, getting 10 minutes here and 10 minutes there, until you've put together 30 minutes during the day. I like to call it "nibbling" on exercise. Use your morning and afternoon breaks and that little time before dinner if you can. It's even been found that fidgeting burns calories. I remember when I was a schoolgirl and the teacher admonished anyone who was swinging his or her legs, saying they weren't concentrating. Little did that teacher know that we students were improving the oxygen flow to our brains and burning calories at the same time.

Excuse: I'm just not motivated.

Fact: Go back to Chapter 13 and read through the stages of change. Maybe you're not ready to change. When you are, the motivation will be there.

Excuse: There aren't any exercise facilities near me.

Fact: Exercise doesn't have to be done in a health club. A good brisk walk or bicycling around your neighborhood is just fine. Go to the mall before it opens (most malls now offer people the opportunity to come in early) and do the "mall walk," brisk walking without window-shopping. If you want exercise that includes instruction (such as aerobics or Pilates, a nonimpact type of exercise), look for some good exercise videos at the store that you can use at home. What about a team sport? Get a group of friends together for a game of ball or Frisbee.

Excuse: It costs too much money.

Fact: You don't have to belong to a health club or spa to exercise, nor do you have to own expensive workout clothes or equipment. The only thing you need is a good pair of athletic shoes.

Excuse: I feel self-conscious.

Fact: Until you get down to a size you feel more comfortable with, a T-shirt with plenty of room to move in should hide whatever part of you that you don't want to share. Keep in mind that your health is at stake and there are others in the same boat.

Excuse: It's too hard.

Fact: Watch a little baby learning to walk and you'll get a feel for how you should approach exercise. A toddler tries a couple of steps and may fall down or intentionally sit down. He or she waits a couple of minutes and then tries again. Never exercise at a level that will cause you pain. However, it won't be very effective if you don't push or exert yourself beyond what's easy.

Excuse: I'm afraid I'll hurt myself.

Fact: Select an activity that feels comfortable for you. Then work your way up gradually to a level you can safely handle. If you're experiencing any pain, you're either not doing the exercise right or it's not right for you.

Excuse: It will make me hungry.

Fact: Actually, exercise helps slow the movement of food through the digestive tract. Glucose is pulled out of the liver into the bloodstream to feed the muscles and, in so doing, helps maintain a more even blood sugar level. That, in turn, should keep you from getting hungry.

An excuse is usually someone's way of saying "I don't want to." Well, if that's true of you, it's your health. However, you couldn't ask for a healthier or quicker way to lose weight. Many people have tried to lose weight by eating fewer calories. That does work to some extent, but not nearly as quickly or effectively as when you include regular exercise. In addition, just eating fewer calories doesn't give you the energy boost that exercising does. Adding 1 hour of exercise per day to a diet that's been decreased by 500 calories per day can slash in half the number of days it takes to lose 1 pound. So part of the reason to exercise is to lose the weight faster. That sounds like a win-win situation to me.

However, a more important reason to exercise is for all the health benefits it offers:

- Lowers blood pressure
- Lowers LDL cholesterol (the bad stuff)
- Improves HDL cholesterol (the good stuff)
- Boosts the metabolism so the body burns more calories
- Provides better blood sugar control
- Helps curb the appetite
- Tightens and preserves muscles
- Improves bone density when the exercise includes weight-bearing activities
- Enhances mood and self-confidence
- Increases energy and productivity
- Improves mental performance
- Provides for a better night's sleep
- Reduces stress and anxiety
- Helps maintain the weight loss

When you think about all the benefits of exercise, it makes you wonder why people aren't finding excuses to get out of doing other things so they can find time to exercise! Before you start an exercise program, though, I'd advise that you check with your doctor first, especially for those of you who are not currently active and might have a health condition.

The Making of a Couch Potato

Considering that the first Olympic Games date back to the eighth century B.C.E., one could assume that exercise and physical prowess have probably always been an important part of the human race. Obviously, even cave dwellers needed to be in good shape if they were going to rustle up some dinner. However, according to a study conducted by the Center for Disease Control, in 2002 only 35.7 percent of male baby boomers did leisure-time physical activity. Female baby boomers came in at an even lower rate of 30.6 percent. So how is it that we have become such couch potatoes? I think it's because we have it too easy. We can drive to the supermarket for our meals—no traditional hunting and gathering necessary. We don't even walk to the market, which many boomer parents did. We eat out quite often, and there's so much prepared food at the market that there's not much physical labor in cooking many of our meals. We do as much as possible with a machine, whether it's cleaning our clothes in a washing machine, washing our dishes in a dishwasher, cutting our grass with a power lawnmower, or whatever. Being an affluent society has probably helped to make this all possible. Don't get me wrong. I'm not saying that we should give up all these amenities, but it does make you realize that we're going to have to figure out another way to burn up calories. Of course, you can always go back to washing your clothes by hand!

Where there's an opportunity, leave it to the manufacturers to provide products to make getting into shape easier for us. An ad for an electrical muscle stimulator states that you can get "six-pack abs electronically" without breaking a sweat. The idea behind the gadget is the use of an electrical current to stimulate the muscle to contract. All you have to do is attach electrodes to various points on your body, turn on the machine, and let it do its wonders. The machine has been used in the medical field to help patients who have muscle problems. It's original intent was not for overweight people. Even though overweight people might get stronger muscles with it, as long as they have a fat layer over the muscles, they'll never see their "washboard" abs. The person still has to lose the weight and the fat. As the saying goes, "There is no free lunch."

Hula hoops were popular when we were younger. While we kids were playing outside with them, our parents were using them indoors for waist reduction. Unfortunately, many adults, who might not have been as coordinated as us kids, threw their backs out. Then there are the treadmills, rowing machines, and exercise bicycles that people buy with the best of intentions. Yet, if you visit garage sales, you'll see many of those good intentions being sold for pennies on the dollar. If you have any of these pieces of exercise equipment in your attic or basement, why not dust them off and see whether you can make them a regular part of your day? If you don't own one and would like to get one, don't bother paying retail when you can buy someone's "best intentions" so cheaply at one of those garage sales.

Making Exercise Fun

For some people, being told to exercise is like being told to eat liver (that is, unless you enjoy liver). All they can picture is suffering, sweating, feeling embarrassed to wear a leotard or shorts, and feeling out of place. If you go to a gym, whom do you watch? Is it the folks who are struggling to get up to speed or the experts, the ones who make it look so easy? Do you realize that watching the experts with envy is no different from plopping a five-year-old into a high school class and expecting him to perform like those students? Remember, everyone crawls before walking.

Watch kids at play. Do you think they ever stop to think about whether they're sweating or getting dirty, or worry about having scratched their knee? They're having fun. That, I believe, is the bottom line for making exercise a part of your life—it should be fun and enjoyable.

Look at the following table and decide what activity would be appealing to you. Some people enjoy an organized activity or a team sport, whereas others would prefer to do their own thing. At the end of the table, I've included some ways you can burn a few extra calories without even trying. Remember, every little bit helps. Whenever I'm asked what exercise I would recommend, I always say, "The one you're willing to do consistently."

Getting Active

Exercise Intensity	Activity
Active	Bicycling, racing Jogging/running, competitive Skiing, cross-country Soccer Stair climbing
Moderate	Aerobic dance Basketball Bicycling, leisurely Ice skating Jogging, leisurely Skiing, downhill

Exercise Intensity	Activity
	Swimming, crawl Tennis, singles Volleyball Walking, briskly
Light	Baseball Gardening Housework Table tennis Tennis, doubles Walking, leisurely
Sedentary	Knitting Typing Playing cards
The Little Extras Count	Put away the television remote and get up to change the channels Use the stairs whenever possible instead of elevators or escalators Park your car far away from your destination Walk to lunch Use a hand-mower to cut your grass instead of a power mower Put a little extra stretch when you vacuum Get a portable phone and walk around as you talk Do some stretching exercises while you watch the microwave cook your food

The Power of Three

If you want to be physically fit, you need to think AFS—**A**erobics, **F**lexibility and **S**trength training.

Aerobic exercise, such as jogging or swimming, is what most people think of as exercise. Flexibility and strength training are seen either as extras or for those interested in becoming bodybuilders. Not so. AFS is a complete package. When you do aerobic exercise, you build stamina, increase lung capacity, strengthen your heart muscle so that it works more efficiently, and get many of the benefits I listed previously.

Look at the table again. If you want to burn fat, it's best to select an aerobic exercise from the Moderate level of activity. The Active level actually uses up more glucose, which is stored in the muscles for energy, instead of relying as heavily on fat cells. And because fat is something you want to get rid of, it's best to do an activity that feeds off of it. Another consideration is the length of time or *duration* of each exercise session and the *frequency* or how many days a week you do it. If you haven't been exercising, then I suggest you start with 20 minutes 3 to 4 times the first week. (You might want to try an exercise from the Light activity level just to get your body used to exercising without too much strain.) Increase your time to 30 minutes 4 or 5 times during the second week. By the third week, go for 40 minutes and consider increasing the *intensity* to a moderate level of activity. At the end of a month, either increase your time per session to 60 minutes or increase the number of days per week you exercise. You can always divide up the time, doing some of your exercise in the morning and some in the evening. Consider doing a variety of activities, because each may contribute differently to your overall fitness.

A great way to determine whether you're exercising at the optimal intensity is to keep track of your heart rate. To find your pulse on your wrist, use your index and middle fingers placed below your thumb of the opposite hand. You can also find the pulse of the carotid artery on your neck, if you prefer. (Sometimes it takes a couple of seconds to locate just the right spot.) Count the number of beats that occur during a 10-second interval. Then multiply that number by six. Now you have your *resting heart rate* per minute.

Your *exercise heart rate zone* is determined based on your age and intensity of exercise. First, subtract your age from 220 to find your *maximum heart rate*. (For example, if you're 45 years old, your maximum heart rate is 175; that is, 220 – 45 = 175.) For the lower end of the heart rate zone, multiply your maximum heart rate by 0.6 (175 × 0.6 = 105). For the upper end, multiply your maximum heart rate by 0.85 (175 × 0.85 = 149). The 45-year-old in this example has established his or her exercise zone—105 to 149 beats per minute.

When you're exercising, monitor your heart rate on your wrist or carotid artery. It should be somewhere between the lower and upper range of your exercise heart rate zone. Remember what I mentioned earlier: A more moderate activity level burns more fat. So if you want, calculate that number by multiplying your maximum heart rate by 70 to 75 percent (0.7 to 0.75). If it makes you feel any better, the older you get, the lower the number can be.

Whenever you complete your exercise session, remember to do at least a five-minute cool-down session. This is the time to slow your activity—walk at a relaxing rate, to keep the blood from pooling in your legs and to give your breathing a chance to return to normal.

I received a joke recently in my e-mail that I just had to share.

An overweight woman goes to see her doctor for him to put her on a diet. The doctor recommends that she eat regularly for two days, then skip a day, and repeat the procedure for two weeks. He told her that she should probably lose at least 5 pounds by her next visit if she followed his instructions.

When the woman returns for her next appointment, she's lost nearly 20 pounds.

"Why that's amazing!" the doctor says. "Did you follow my instructions?"

The woman nods and says, "I'll tell you, though, I thought I was going to drop dead on the third day."

"From hunger, you mean?" asked the doctor.

"No, from all that skipping," she replied.

Flexibility exercises, such as calisthenics, martial arts, tai chi, and yoga, consist of stretching all parts of your body. Flexibility is probably the most overlooked part of an exercise program. Yet it's really one of the most important. You want your muscles to flex with motion like a reed in the wind. If they don't, you run a higher risk of hurting yourself, losing your balance, or worse, breaking something. Besides, there's such a great feeling when you're in the slow process of a stretch, feeling the muscle lengthen.

I can speak from experience. My hamstrings were so short that I had a hard time bending over to touch my toes. So I started doing some stretching exercises. At first, I was very discouraged, because it seemed like I was going nowhere fast. (You can't be impatient with flexibility exercises. You must let the muscle stretch at its own pace.) However, as I continued diligently every morning for about 20 minutes, I finally started seeing some results. First it only seemed like millimeters. Then it started feeling like inches. Now I can even do a spread eagle and can almost touch my chest to the floor.

I suggest that you don't look in a mirror as you do stretching exercises. Feel the muscle and follow its lead. When you're looking in a mirror, you may push further to reach a particular position, even though the muscle isn't ready to go that far. You may end up hurting yourself.

Last is **strength training.** Lifting weights, using resistance equipment, or even using your own body weight (such as with crunches or sit-ups) encourages the building of muscle. One thing I don't think most people appreciate is that weak stomach muscles can lead to back problems. Those "abs of steel" people strive for aren't just for looks. Keep in mind that muscle burns more calories than fat cells. So it just makes sense to build as much muscle as you can. I'm not suggesting that you bulk up like greased bodybuilders. (Of course, if you get yourself that committed to building that much muscle mass, I won't worry about your losing weight.)

It's encouraging to know that there are studies that show you can increase muscle at any age. Hooray, we boomers still have a chance! If you go to a gym or read a book on exercise, you'll discover such terms as *frequency, resistance,* and *repetitions.* A good starter frequency for strength training would be three days a week. The resistance refers to the number of pounds in the weights or tension you use, and repetitions (reps) are the number of times you perform a particular exercise. It's better to start with lighter weights and do more reps. If you hurt yourself at the beginning, you're not going to want, or possibly even be able, to continue.

Strength training and aerobic exercises that are weight bearing also help strengthen bones. Bones are living tissue, with calcium constantly flowing back and forth between the bone and the blood. Exercise that creates an impact with the ground encourages calcium to flow into the bones. Most aerobic exercises are weight bearing. Swimming is not weight bearing, even though it is a great aerobic sport.

As I've been sharing with you the types of exercise that would make your body happy and healthy, have you been wondering how you could ever fit all that exercise into a week? It sounds overwhelming if you think you have to do it all at one time. You don't have to. First, determine whether exercising before you go to work or get your day started is doable. It may mean that you need to get up about 30 to 40 minutes earlier than normal to do some aerobic exercise. Look at this as a great way to wake up all the cells in your body, getting your blood flowing and oxygen to your brain. Are you willing to do that? If you feel you can only spare 20 minutes in the morning, do some flexibility or strength training. When you get home from work, do the aerobic exercise.

Let's do some brainstorming here. I've created a schedule for the person who can dedicate about 20 minutes in the morning to some exercise, but needs to save the afternoon or evening for the longer bouts of aerobic exercise. Does this look like it could work for you? If not, create a schedule that will.

Exercise	Monday	Tuesday	Wednesday	Thursday	Friday	Saturday	Sunday
Aerobic	P.M.	P.M.		P.M.	P.M.	P.M.	P.M.
Flexibility	A.M.		A.M.		A.M.		
Strength		A.M.		A.M.		P.M.	

If you haven't been an exerciser, then you're going to have to be a person who "believes before you see." It takes time for the body to respond, but once it does, then "seeing is believing."

In Appendix K, I've included an exercise log you can use to keep track of your AFS. To get more ideas on great exercises, you might want to read *Body for Life,* by Bill Phillips.

Bite-Size Advice

Forget the "no pain, no-gain" philosophy. It doesn't make any sense to do something that hurts (unless you're a masochist!). When you're hurt, you can't do anything good for yourself.

Take small steps in adding exercise to your daily routine. Increase your level of activity as your body adjusts. Try using a pedometer as both a monitor of how many steps you take during the day and as a way to goal-set. If you took 1,000 steps today, try for 200 more tomorrow and 300 more the next day.

To get physical doesn't mean you have to be involved in a regimented exercise program. Just taking a walk, dancing, or even shopping—to name a few activities—will keep you active without requiring much structure.

Exercise is a great mood enhancer and stress reducer. Use exercise after work as a way to unwind before dinner. It even helps control your appetite.

Replace some of your motorized equipment with a manual model. Use a push-style lawnmower instead of your power mower; use a shovel instead of your snow blower.

Be consistent by exercising on a regular basis. Exercising every day is optimal. But if you can't do that, then at least shoot for five times per week. Don't be a "weekend warrior," trying to fit in four or five days' worth of exercise in one or two days. That's not how your body likes it—and it'll tell you so.

Make an appointment with exercise. Put it on your calendar for specific days and times each week. And you don't get to cancel your appointments unless it's absolutely necessary (and, oh yes, you have to have a note from your mother!).

Make the most of your time. Listen to books on tape or set up your exercise environment so that you can watch television as you exercise.

Don't forget to drink plenty of fluids. That applies before, during, and after you exercise.

Choose a type of exercise that you enjoy. If you do an exercise that's "good for you," but brings you no pleasure, you probably won't continue with it for long. Remember, the objective of this book is to help you find what's comfortable for you to do as part of a permanent lifestyle.

Sometimes just getting started is the hardest part. Tell yourself that you only need to exercise for five minutes. If, after five minutes, you can't get through it, you can quit. However, I think you'll find that, after getting into the right attire, putting your shoes on and getting out the front door, you'll become committed. You just needed to get to that point.

Maybe add a little element of competition to your exercise regimen. Call on a friend to be your competitor. See who can exercise most frequently, stay on track longest, or reach their goal soonest.

Exercise in the morning before you head off to work. Who knows what will happen after work that'll interfere with your best of intentions.

Don't expect overnight results. It may take up to six weeks for your body to adjust to the new level of activity and for your fat cells to give up their most treasured possession—fat. Don't forget that muscle weighs more than fat. With all the exercise you're hopefully doing, you'll be increasing your muscle and decreasing your fat. It may take a little while for the scale to reflect the new you. However, look in the mirror. Those tighter abdominal muscles and buttocks should be evidence enough.

chapter 30

Diet Tips for Smaller Hips

I'd do anything to look like him, except exercise and eat right.

—Steve Martin

Whether you're a Planner or Ad-libber, use the tips in this chapter as you would one-a-day vitamins. Read one tip a day, and see how it works for you. Some tips are suggestions of things to try, and others are more like did-you-know type of messages. You don't have to take your one-a-day tips in order. Maybe quickly read through them. Then go back and each day select one that sounds interesting to you to try.

Basic Tips

Remember the KISS rule. When what you're doing to lose weight seems too complicated, it's probably the wrong thing to do. If nothing else, it certainly isn't something you're going to do indefinitely. So the best rule of thumb is **K**eep **I**t **S**uper **S**imple.

Preview, do, review. This is another good rule to keep in mind. In the morning, before you jump out of bed, preview your day. Think about what you're going to do to stick to your weight-loss goals, what might be some of the challenges you'll face, and how you might plan on handling them. During the day, do the eating plan you've selected, remembering the thoughts you previewed. At the end of the day, before you fall asleep, review what happened during the day. Were you able to stick to your plan? If not, what got in the way and how did you handle it? For those of you who find keeping records a way to stay on task, create a Preview, Do, Review Log. At the end of each week, re-read what you've written and see what's working and what's not.

Be realistic. Because gaining the extra weight didn't happen overnight, losing it overnight won't happen either. Try making small changes that over time can realistically be achieved. Don't set your goal weight so low that it'll be impossible to reach. Consider what's reasonable.

Be flexible. Appreciate that every day isn't going to be perfect. Allow that slips are going to happen (as long as there aren't too many of them!). What's more important is how you handle the slip.

Make a list of obstacles. Write down barriers you think you might encounter while losing weight. Next to each item, write down something you can do that will neutralize or eliminate that challenge.

Burn more calories than you consume. No matter what eating plan you follow, losing weight boils down to this.

Cinch your belt. Make it one notch tighter when you sit down to eat. You'll have a constant reminder of when to stop eating.

Don't make excuses. There's no good reason for eating poorly or for not exercising. Don't try to rationalize an irrational behavior. It won't get you any closer to your goal.

Focus on your successes. Concentrate on your accomplishments rather than on your failures. When you put too much attention on where you've failed, you lose track of where you're going.

"All-or-nothing thinking" can be your undoing. Just because you think you blew your weight-loss efforts by eating a piece of candy doesn't mean you get to eat the rest of the box. Or maybe you've lost five pounds, but put two of them back on. So what? Avoid this kind of all-or-nothing, win-or-lose thinking that says, "You're a failure, so you might as well go back to your old ways. This way doesn't work."

Be honest with yourself. Decide what you really believe you're capable of doing. Although I believe everyone can stretch a little, you shouldn't go too far beyond what's comfortable. After all, a rubber band that's stretched too far will break.

Progress, not perfection. That's the name of the game.

When you look in the mirror, what do you see? The image you perceive is more a reflection of what you think about yourself than what's actually there. For example, after you've eaten healthfully and exercised for a couple of days, there probably won't be a lot of physical change. Yet, somehow you see a different you. Remember how that feels the next time you look in the mirror and say something derogatory, such as "I look horrible today" or "I'm such a blimp." Would you call a friend or loved one names like that? Then why do it to yourself?

Well-rested people eat less. People who are tired or who've been deprived of sleep tend to reach for sugary foods, thinking that these foods will energize them. Yet just the opposite happens, because of the effect sugar has on their blood level of glucose and their insulin response. A better choice than snacking is to get a good night's rest, to take a quick nap, or maybe to take a short walk.

Don't give up. Sometimes the struggle is not in changing your lifestyle habits, but getting others to accept that you're doing something good for yourself. Don't listen to what others say. When you do arrive at your goal weight, their tone will change and compliments will abound.

Avoid generalizing. Just because you were unsuccessful on the last two diets doesn't mean that the same thing will happen on this one. Part of the reason is that this time you're not going on a diet. You're learning to do something good for yourself that you'll do for the rest of your life.

Don't be a "shoulda-coulda-woulda" person. So you didn't eat as well as you could have or you didn't exercise when you should have. Move past the mistake, using it as a learning experience.

Goal-set "through" rather than "to" the weight you want to be. It's interesting how many people lose their drive and motivation the closer they get to their goal weight. Some people believe that "reaching the goal" means they can stop whatever they were doing to get there.

In the case of losing weight, "setting a goal through," unlike dieting, means you have to continue your new lifestyle in order to maintain the loss.

Eliminate stinkin' thinkin'. Remember, you're not on a diet; you're eating healthfully and exercising.

Weigh yourself once a week, at most. The bathroom scale can be a useful tool in losing weight when it's used properly. Weigh yourself the same day of the week, at the same time (preferably in the morning, right after you get up and have gone to the bathroom), and without your clothes on. A scale is not a mood meter. Don't look at your weight on the scale to determine what kind of attitude you're going to have the rest of the day!

Alternative-to-eating list. Create some ready options to do when you're about to go for food or find yourself eating even though you're not actually hungry. If you're bored, frustrated, anxious, or whatever, call a friend, take a walk, write a letter, listen to music, read a book, take a bubble bath.

Analyze your cravings. Is it the particular food you're craving or the contentment it brings? (Stress may be your problem.) Maybe cookies or ice cream comforted you in the past, when life seemed to be going wrong, and now something's happening that makes you feel the same way. A better alternative might be an aerobic workout that helps send comforting endorphins through your system.

Healthy Eating Tips

Be adventurous. Try new foods and different types of physical activity to make the process more interesting. Don't wait until you've reached your goal to really live life. Remember, life is a journey.

Be sensible. Saying "I'm never going to eat cake again" is unreasonable. The only place for "never" is in the story of Peter Pan and Never-Never Land. Whereas you should enjoy what you eat or what you do for exercise, just don't overdo it. It's not that different from driving a car. When you're behind the wheel on the freeway, only small adjustments need to be made in your steering to stay within the lines—so, too, with your eating or exercising. To drastically cut your calories or excessively exercise is like adjusting your steering so you're swerving from lane to lane in an attempt to actually stay in the center of the lane. Moderation is the key.

Eat as if you're being watched. If someone were there watching you, would you "sneak" food? Would you stuff food into your mouth, taking more than you can easily chew? How about eating the food off someone else's plate on its way to the sink? Would you polish off an entire container of ice cream? I doubt whether you'd do these things openly and consciously. So next time, let your conscience be your guide. Make believe someone is watching you—*you*.

Think substitution, not addition. You may want to add something that's healthy to your plate, but are you going to end up with too much food? If so, remove something that's not so healthy to make room. Or reduce the quantity of everything. Don't eat more calories than you need, justifying it by saying "but I'm eating this healthy item, too."

Good diets and bad diets. You may think that there are good foods and bad foods, but that's not the case. Instead of considering an individual food, consider what you eat in the context of the whole day or several days.

Don't eat "your last supper." Don't "pig out" before you start on your weight-loss journey because you think you'll never get to eat "those foods" again. Remember, there are no bad foods, just bad weight-loss approaches. All foods are legal unless you've been told to avoid certain ones by your doctor.

Forget the notion of "eating for later." Stuffing yourself at a meal so you won't be hungry in a couple of hours doesn't work. Oftentimes, the more food you eat, the faster you rev up your metabolism. Then you end up being just as hungry, or more so, four hours later as you would have been had you eaten just enough to satisfy your appetite.

Foods that trigger eating for you may be best kept out of the house. Identify the items that you can't resist. Is it nuts? Chips? Ice cream? You might be better off not having them in your house. When you really want them, go out to enjoy them.

Eating should not be a transition activity. For example, you've just come home from work and stop by the pantry to grab a cookie on your way to changing your clothes. Why? If you weren't hungry, you've picked up a very bad habit. If you are hungry, then learn to sit down and eat. Eating should not be a way of taking care of boredom, frustration, and anger. Nor should it be a means of avoiding doing something else.

Stock your pantry with healthy foods. Try to keep "risky" foods—the ones you know you could pig out on given the chance—out of the house. Save them for special occasions. Instead, buy healthy alternatives that don't cause you guilt when you eat them.

Taste satisfaction without all the calories. Ice cream doesn't have to be eaten out of a dish or a cone. To get enjoyment without all the calories, scoop just 1 spoonful out of the container and *immediately* put the container back in the freezer. Then slowly lick the spoon to make the pleasure last.

You can "have your cake and eat it, too." Just make sure it's not on the same day you're having a cheeseburger, fries, and a shake. It doesn't have to be the whole slice, either.

Have a cup of hot broth. About 20 minutes before each meal, have a cup of hot broth or about 4 ounces of vegetable juice. This announces to your body and mind that food is soon on its way. It should keep you from eating ravenously on anything that's at hand.

Don't skip meals or snacks. Otherwise, you may overeat the next time you have contact with food. By eating each meal, you're less likely to experience cravings. Most importantly, don't skip breakfast. Breakfast is really the most important meal of the day. It literally means "break the fast." You haven't eaten since dinner the night before. By eating breakfast, you jump-start your metabolism for the day and are less likely to grab a high-fat, high-calorie pastry at midmorning. Your performance for the day will be much improved.

Eat stronger flavors. You may end up eating less food because your taste buds have been well satisfied. Blander foods may cause you to eat more. So for example, eat blue cheese instead of havarti cheese.

Water is as important to your health as the food you eat. Try to drink about 8 glasses a day. For those of you who can't imagine drinking that much, try the following. Fill a half-gallon container with water and put it in the refrigerator. Challenge yourself to see how much of it you can drink throughout the day. Each day start again, seeing whether you can drink more than the previous day. Before you know it, you'll be drinking 8 glasses easily.

Eat because you're hungry, not because you're thirsty. A glass of water or juice may be all you need.

Consider fat a flavoring. Don't think of it as a food.

Keep hard candies handy. When you have a craving for something sweet, slowly suck (do not chew!) to satisfy that sweet tooth.

Give up the "clean-your-plate" syndrome. This is probably something you developed in childhood, when your mother told you to eat everything in front of you because of all the starving children in the world. Now that you're an adult, I hope you've learned that stuffing yourself will not do those children any good. Learn to leave a little food on your plate.

Quality not quantity. Eating a piece of luxurious rich dark chocolate very slowly, to enjoy all of its flavor nuances, may be much more satisfying than eating a whole bag of cheap waxy chocolate (and much less fattening).

Spend your calories wisely. Select foods you really enjoy rather than wasting your calories on "just anything." Although you should eat healthfully, you should also enjoy what you eat.

Eat what you like. Otherwise, you're going to feel deprived—and then, watch out. You'll find yourself binging and overindulging on high-fat/high-calorie foods to make up for it. If it's something that's fattening or full of calories, just eat less. Thinking you can fill up on celery sticks when what you really wanted was a piece of chocolate isn't going to work.

Cravings do pass. Believe it or not. They're like a wave on the ocean, building and building until it crashes on the shore. But have you been at the beach and noticed that a wave, once it has crashed, quietly retreats back into the ocean? The same is true with a craving. If you'll just hold off on that urge for about 10 to 15 minutes, you'll find that its strength and its hold on you will retreat just like the wave. Most importantly, don't focus on the craving. Find a distraction—watch television, watch people, read a book, work on a puzzle, play a game, call a friend, organize your closets and drawers, go shopping.

Sit down. Whenever you eat, whether it's a snack or a meal, sit down and take note of what you're eating. In other words, no eating on the run or standing in front of the refrigerator!

Slow down. Eat slowly so you give the food time to pass through your stomach and into your intestines. It's there that the message "we're finally getting fed" is sent to your brain. Because it takes about 20 minutes for all this to happen, you can imagine how much extra food you can eat before the message is received when you eat too quickly.

Don't be distracted while eating. If I were to ask you an hour after you finished eating what you'd had, would you be able to tell me? Too many people eat while doing something else, like reading or watching television, or getting into heated debates. They hardly notice what they've eaten (or how much). If you're going to eat—whether it's just a snack or a complete meal—enjoy it, savor the flavors, make the process special.

Plate size. Serve your meal on a salad plate instead of a dinner plate.

Eat your vegetables first. Before you fill up on the other parts of your meal, eat your vegetables so the bulk will give you a full feeling and might help you avoid overeating.

Be consistent. After you've established a healthy way of eating that feels comfortable for you, keep it up.

Brush your teeth. If you brush immediately after you finish eating the main course, but before dessert, you might find yourself skipping those extra calories. That's because brushing your teeth will leave a sufficiently pleasant flavor in your mouth to make the dessert course unnecessary. Besides, when your mouth feels fresh and clean, you're less likely to put more food in it.

Don't use food as a reward. When you're doing well with your weight-loss efforts, you deserve to be rewarded, just not with food. How about getting yourself a massage? A new outfit? See a special show? You might even consider putting a dollar bill in a jar each time you've reached a certain milestone and when enough money accumulates, take a vacation.

Focus. Think about the foods you should be eating rather than on the foods you think you should be avoiding. That way you won't constantly feel you're being deprived. It just won't be on your mind.

Try grazing. Instead of having just three big meals a day, have some of your breakfast foods for a midmorning snack. Save something from lunch and eat as your midafternoon snack. Instead of eating dessert right after dinner, eat it a little while before you go to bed. The advantage of grazing is that it keeps your blood sugar at a more constant level, rather than rising up and falling like a roller-coaster ride.

Chew, chew, chew. When eating solid foods, chew them well and don't use liquids to swallow them down. When you use liquids, you're probably eating too quickly and not getting as much mouth pleasure as you could. By spending more time chewing your food, the saliva that you work up should be enough to help the food glide down.

A Little Humor for Encouragement

Is it true that when someone doesn't see you eating, the calories don't count?

Why do people always twist open an Oreo cookie before eating it? That's to let the calories fall out.

Food that is eaten standing up only gets your feet fat because gravity causes those calories to end up there.

Popcorn and candy eaten at the movies don't count because they're part of the complete entertainment package.

Clever way to look thinner: Stay around people who are fatter.

Foods of the same color have the same number of calories. So mint chocolate chip ice cream is equivalent to spinach? Or white chocolate is equivalent to cauliflower?

The calories in a candy bar are cancelled out by drinking a diet soda.

Foods used for medicinal purposes, such as hot chocolate or hot buttered rum, don't count.

Ingredients eaten while preparing a dish don't have any calories because they're not yet part of the finished dish.

When your talking bathroom scale says "one at a time," you know it's time to lose weight.

Calories are a measure of how good a food tastes. Take fudge, for example.

chapter 31

Mind Your Mood

Life is what happens while you are busy making other plans.
—John Lennon

I saved this chapter on mood for the end, because, for many people, that's where becoming overweight begins. If food was used to pacify you when you were younger, do you still use food to handle stress? When you do, does the food just distract you or does it actually make you feel better? We'll explore that concept in a moment. But before we do, keep in mind that using food as a stress reliever is not an effective approach. Here's why. Considering the physiology of stress, it's interesting that some people should turn to food at a time when they're feeling stressed out. All the chemistry that's going on in the body during a stressful incident isn't conducive to efficient food digestion. Even though you may not realize it, every time you experience stress, your body is going through a "fight-or-flight" reaction. The degree of the reaction may vary depending upon the situation, but the same body chemistry happens just the same.

Imagine that you're walking alone on a deserted street (not something I recommend) and you notice a scruffy bearded man in tattered clothes coming out of a doorway. He starts to follow you. Your pulse begins to quicken. You pick up your pace, and he does, too. Is this just a coincidence? What does he want? Your mind starts creating images of what he could do to you. The next thing you know you're running for safety. The adrenaline is pumping. Blood is being directed to your legs and heart to provide the maximum amount of oxygen and energy to help you get away. Your heart rate, blood pressure, breathing, and metabolism have increased. Is this the time you'd like to have a full stomach from a big meal? No! Then why eat at times of mental stress?

Under normal circumstances, after you eat, there is increased blood flow to the stomach and digestive tract to facilitate digestion. However, in the frightful situation just described, that blood is not going to be available to your stomach—it's being diverted to your legs and heart. The food in your stomach will just have to sit there, potentially causing distress, until much later when all the fight-or-flight chemicals have subsided. (Think about an athlete. He or she doesn't eat a big meal before a competition for just this reason.)

Now consider that, instead of being chased by someone, you've just had an argument with a loved one. You'll get the same fight-or-flight physiological response. Your body's reaction is no different. Your heart rate, breathing, and metabolism increase. In fact, the fight-or-flight response can happen no matter how big or small the event. Just someone cutting in front of you on the freeway can get your system riled up. Or how about the person who got the parking space you had your eye on? And what about the IRS, which just sent you a notice that they plan to audit you? So how do you deal with these life stresses? Will you comfort yourself by eating something—your usual response? If you do, please remember that your blood isn't going to be there to digest what you just ate, because you've got a fight-or-flight reaction in progress.

Looking to food to comfort you isn't going to work. Because digestion has slowed or completely come to a halt, whatever you ate isn't going to get into your system until long after the crisis has past. Then why are you eating it? If you're hoping that that chocolate candy will make things "all better," it won't. If it's to distract you from the incident, there are far healthier ways. Go take a walk or jog. Call a friend and get what's on your chest off. Work on a fun project. If you have to involve your mouth in some way, you'd be better off chewing gum or even sucking on a baby pacifier. (I won't tell.) At least it's better than chewing on pencils and eating lead.

Lack of control over a situation can be a major contributor to stress in our lives. Being told what to do, or feeling you can't change anything, makes you want to turn to what you do have control over—food. Worrying about an event or situation in the future is an example of something you don't have control over. Much as you try to plan for the future, only when the future finally becomes the present will you be able to react appropriately. Until then, it's just speculation. I saw a great saying on a porcelain tile that sums it up nicely: "Worry is the misuse of your imagination." Yet even happy events, such as winning the lottery, can be stressful. And what do you do when you win the lottery? Go out to dinner and celebrate. Again, the food is just going to sit there until the rest of your body has had the chance to calm down, which will then allow the food to be digested.

We can't forget the training we had when we were younger—a cookie for what ails you. As adults we've raised the ante—this time it's a pint of ice cream or what's left of the chocolate cake that was just cut into the other night. Worse yet, you may not even be enjoying the food. Remember what I shared with you earlier in the book. You should focus on what you eat and enjoy it. With your mind monopolized by the stressful incident, you can't be thinking about what you're eating. So it's mindless eating. What a waste of calories. It's too easy to forget that food is for sustenance, to make you strong and healthy. To use it for other reasons is to abuse it.

The Food-Mood Connection

Although the title of this section is The Food-Mood Connection, it could just as well have been called The Mood-Food Connection. Your mood can be very much influenced by the food you eat. On the other hand, your mood may dictate the food you want. The former is a *proactive* approach to handling your emotions and well-being, whereas the latter is *reactive*.

So do you want to be more alert and productive, or do you want to be more relaxed and calm? That probably depends upon what time of the day it is and what you need to accomplish. If you have a morning meeting, I'm sure you're going to want to be on your toes and well focused. After work, when you're tired from the day, I'm sure you'd enjoy being able to unwind. And when you go to bed, it would be nice to fall asleep easily, wouldn't it? What you eat can very strongly influence whether you can achieve these states of mind.

Judith J. Wurtman, Ph.D., in her book *Managing Your Mind and Mood Through Food,* shares how the foods you eat can help you improve your performance and deal with stress. Wouldn't we all want to bounce out of bed in the morning and face the day with energy and a great attitude? Getting a good night's sleep is a good start. But then what? First, you need to eat a good breakfast. Many people, especially those who don't really enjoy breakfast, grab a piece of fruit, toast with jam, coffee, and say they've had breakfast. What they just had was a meal to fall asleep on by about midmorning. That's because it was all carbohydrates.

You need to understand how the body deals with the different nutrients so you can have control over the mood state your body ends up in. Once digested and absorbed, carbohydrates and proteins influence the chemicals in your brain. These chemicals, in turn, affect your mood, energy level, and mental alertness. It's great that you can have some control over which of these chemicals is going to be the most active. What did you eat for your last meal? Believe it or not, what you ate is affecting how you feel as you're reading this book. If you're feeling groggy, you've probably just had a good dose of carbohydrates (or, heaven forbid, I'm boring you). If you're alert and can't wait to read more, you probably had a good helping of protein (or, as I hope is the case, you're really enjoying what you're reading).

Let me share with you how this works. There are three major brain chemicals, called *neurotransmitters,* which are involved in mood alteration. They are dopamine, norepinephrine, and serotonin. They serve as messengers between neurons or nerves in your brain, telling them what they need to do. Although these chemicals are always present, the relative quantities of each are based on what you eat or what situation you might find yourself in. Dopamine and norepinephrine are considered the alertness chemicals, whereas serotonin is considered the calming chemical. All three of these chemicals are made from amino acids, the building blocks of proteins. For this discussion, we're only going to be concerned with the amino acids *tyrosine* and *tryptophan*. Tyrosine is a major ingredient in the production of dopamine and norepinephrine. Tryptophan is the major ingredient in making serotonin.

Now here's where you get to be in control. When you need to be alert, say for that afternoon meeting you have scheduled, what neurotransmitters do you want to have plenty of? Dopamine and norepinephrine. And what amino acid do you need to have in rich supply for that to happen? Tyrosine. So what you now need to know is—what are good sources of tyrosine in your diet? The answer is high-protein foods with little fat. Too much fat slows the digestion process, making the necessary amino acid not as readily available. Some actual food suggestions would include chicken, very lean beef, fish, shellfish, low-fat dairy products, legumes and dry beans, tofu, and soy products. A power lunch would be something like a grilled chicken salad or shrimp cocktail. Avoid the starches—you'll soon see why.

Now, imagine that you've had a hard day. Maybe your boss had some choice words with you or your kids wouldn't stop complaining about one thing or another or someone nearly ran you over in the crosswalk. You get the picture. You're tense and irritable. Don't go chowing down on steak. It's time to bring out the pasta, breads, and grains—the "comfort foods." That's because carbohydrates, eaten by themselves without any additional protein (say, in the form of meat), encourages the amino acid tryptophan to enter your brain and stimulate the production of serotonin.

What's interesting is that tyrosine and tryptophan enter your brain through the same doorway. When you have a high-protein meal, you're getting both tyrosine and tryptophan. However, tyrosine, which is a more plentiful amino acid than tryptophan, is pushier and more successful. It's able to shove tryptophan out of the way, so it can get through the entrance to the brain. The brain becomes flooded with plenty of tyrosine to stimulate the production of dopamine and norepinephrine. The result is that you end up more focused, attentive, and, overall, more energetic.

So if tyrosine seems to have the advantage, how can you get tryptophan into your brain when you want a calming effect?

The answer—you need to eat carbohydrates. I told you earlier in the book that when you eat carbohydrates, they're absorbed as glucose and stimulate the pancreas to secrete insulin. Insulin not only helps move glucose into the cells to stabilize your blood sugar, but also encourages proteins to enter various sites throughout the body (such as muscle, bone, and organs). However, tryptophan, even though it's a protein, doesn't readily go into these sites, and so it continues to float around in your bloodstream. When it arrives at your brain, it has less competition getting through the doorway. It can now enter more freely to help create serotonin, the calming chemical.

Knowing how proteins and carbohydrates can affect your mood and performance should help you understand why it's best to eat your protein earlier in the day. You want to be sharp during the day and laid-back at night (that is, unless you have a night job and all of this would be reversed). Most of us grew up with a meat-and-potatoes-style dinner. What made you think you were getting tired was the high fat content of the meal, which slowed down your digestion. But how many times have you had a high-protein dinner and found yourself wide awake when it was time to go to bed? The protein had finally digested, and the tyrosine had gone to work on your brain. It may take a little mind changing to accept having a dinner that's strictly pasta, vegetables, and fruit. However, if you had your protein allowance earlier in the day, what difference would it make if you had a strictly carbohydrate dinner? If dinner for you isn't dinner without meat, just have a small portion, eat a smaller quantity of food, and save some of your carbohydrate allowance for a snack at least an hour before bed.

How many times have you had a piece of candy in the afternoon as a pick-me-up, only to find, not long after, that it ended up being more like a let-me-down? We often think sugar should give us a boost, rationalizing that the reason we're feeling a lack of energy is low blood sugar. In truth, it may actually be an insufficient amount of tyrosine getting to your brain to keep you alert. And please take note that the candy is a carbohydrate, which is going to encourage the production of serotonin.

If you get any energy boost from the candy, it may either be mental or it may be a quick blood sugar rise that isn't going to last long.

Putting It Together

I told you that you really shouldn't eat anything when you're under stress. Emergencies will happen, and you can't prepare for them. But turning to food isn't going to help, because the food isn't going to be digested fast enough to influence your brain chemistry. Learning to do deep-breathing exercises or meditation would have far more value. (And they're not fattening!) They can be done wherever you are, requiring no special equipment or clothing. The only suggestion I'd make, if the situation allowed it, would be to loosen your belt, men loosen your tie, and women loosen your bra.

Learning to breathe deeply would be beneficial, because most of us normally breathe much too shallowly anyway. Why don't you try it? Close your eyes (after you've read the instructions!). Place your hand on your abdomen. Inhale through your nose very slowly to the count of four. Feel your abdomen rise. Hold that for two counts. Then exhale through your mouth, again to the count of four. Your abdomen should contract. Concentrate on the energy being drawn in through your nose, imagining it traveling throughout your body (all the way to your toes). Do this until you feel the tension in your body subside.

If you want to try meditation, the easiest would be the *mantra meditation*. Find a short word that's meaningful to you, or come up with a special sound. A traditional mantra uses the word *om,* where you bring your lips together and allow the word to vibrate in your mouth until it disappears. Focus and concentrate on the sound of the word. If you find your mind wandering, gently bring it back to what you're doing. Continue to do this until you feel your blood pressure getting back to normal.

chapter 32

Make It Last

It's so hard when I have to, and so easy when I want to.

—Sondra Anice Barnes

In the movie *Star Wars: The Empire Strikes Back,* Yoda, the Jedi master, is working with Luke Skywalker to help him become a Jedi warrior. Luke's spacecraft had ended up in a marsh when he landed. His challenge was to figure out how he could get the spacecraft lifted out of the marsh without any equipment. Yoda told Luke that, with the power of the "force," he'd be able to move the spacecraft. Luke responded, "All right. I'll give it a try." To which Yoda replied, "No! Try not. Do, or do not. There is no 'try'."

This quote is very appropriate to your mission of losing weight. If you take what you've read in this book and say, "I'll try it and see," then I suggest you give this book to someone else who's truly committed to making the change happen. Trying means that you're not fully invested in the process and, therefore, you're willing to accept failure. You must *do,* for only by *doing* will you exert all your efforts until you succeed. It may involve your "believing before seeing." But if you wait for "seeing is believing," you won't make it.

Although you do have your work cut out for you, keep remembering that it's for a worthwhile cause—*you.* The suggestions I've made in this book aren't difficult to understand or to follow. The challenge for you will be sticking with it. Most people are excited about getting started and having the opportunity to finally get it right. But that's not what counts. What's really important is having the resolve to do what it takes—not just at the beginning, not just for one time, but until your body accepts its new weight as the new norm. It may require that you give up some of your old ways of doing things and see life from a different perspective. Actually, when you think about it, that shouldn't be so hard, considering the fact that what you've been doing hasn't been working anyway. So embracing a new way of dealing with life may be the answer.

Think about Ebenezer Scrooge in Charles Dickens's *A Christmas Carol.* Had he not been visited by the three ghosts—that of Christmas Past, Christmas Present, and Christmas Yet to Come—he might never have realized the error of his ways—and what his life was leading him to. You, too, need to visit your past and present dietary and life patterns, and look ahead to where they might be leading you. As Scrooge was told by the spirit of Christmas Yet to Come, he could make changes now that would alter what might be. Scrooge was willing to change, saying, "I will not shut out the lessons that they teach." I hope that that will be true for you, as well.

One of the qualities of happiness is optimism. Optimism gives you the power to believe you can do it; that all you've gone through to get you to this point are lessons for you to use going forward; that you needn't fear your future because you have a chance to change and influence that future.

Happiness comes from being healthy. To be healthy requires that you take control of your life, rather than letting life control you. Always remember that you have a choice. You have the freedom to decide what to eat, when to exercise, and how to deal with stress. When you realize that you have the personal power to be the best you can be, you will be. That's the strength of the human character—to rise above it all, despite the odds. If you've lost weight before and gained it back, you may believe the odds are against you—you may figure that you probably won't be successful this time either. I'd like to think otherwise. You've got the tools to lose weight in your hands right now—not only in this book; but in your self. You weaken yourself to think otherwise. It's like Samson thinking he lost his strength when his hair was cut.

The Choice Is Yours

As boomers, we're old enough to have experienced a good deal of life so far, becoming wiser every year (I hope!). There are few people who aren't truly aware of the dangers of being overweight. It's almost embarrassing to say, "I didn't know." Not to address the problem is just being an ostrich, hiding your head in the sand.

> *Advice is what we ask for when we already know the answer but wish we didn't.*
>
> —*Erica Jong*

Does it come down to deciding between *quality* versus *quantity* of life? I'd like to think you can have them both.

Defining quantity of life is pretty straightforward. I want as many years as I can get on this planet. In fact, let me be the one to set the old-age record! With all the medical advances that have been made during our lifetime, we boomers have a chance of setting new longevity records. But we'll never get there if we don't take care of the obesity problem that's running rampant in the United States. We know that the risk for heart disease, diabetes, and some cancers are increased by obesity. These devastating diseases aren't to be taken lightly. Do you realize how many things you fix when you lose weight? You decrease your risk for disease, become more energetic, have an easier time moving, put less strain on your joints, look better in your clothes, feel better about yourself, and so on. Is there anything else that you do in your life that is as rewarding?

Quality of life, on the other hand, is harder to identify. It means something different for each person. For some, being able to eat all the hamburgers and soda they want, and never having to sweat over some exercise regimen, defines quality of life. For them, it's not having to give anything up, nor even caring to think about the consequences of living life that way. They'll never succeed at losing weight and keeping it off. A person like this hasn't established a healthy relationship with food. Although I believe that you should enjoy food, the reason for eating is to nourish your body. Try to take note of when it feels that food has taken on a life of its own—making itself master over you. Some people would like to say that cravings just show that you need certain nutrients. If you think that may be true for you, take a multivitamin with minerals that contains no more than 100% Daily Value for each of the nutrients and see the results. More than likely, previous experiences with certain foods, and just plain habit, have created a dependency.

Think about how you establish a healthy relationship with a person. First you meet. Then you get to know each other. Only after you've found that you have enough in common do you pursue a deeper relationship. The same thing can apply to food. Try something new. Cook it in various ways to see how you like it. If it's something you enjoy, then it may become a permanent part of your menu. On the flip side are the foods that get you into trouble. People sometimes choose to get a divorce because of irreconcilable differences—maybe you need to divorce yourself from the foods that are unhealthy and controlling you. Don't bring them into the house or expose yourself to them.

> Mr. Jones goes to the doctor and says, "Doc, it hurts when I move my arm this way." To which the doctor replies, "Then don't move it that way."
>
> Moral of the joke: You're in control—as long as you take control.

For those of you who view quality of life as looking good, feeling good, and having so much energy that you never feel old, you need to do what it takes to achieve it. And, by the way, if you're willing to do what it takes, you probably have a good shot at quantity of life, as well. It doesn't hurt to have some relatives in your family who have lived to a ripe old age, but even if you don't, why can't you be the one to start the trend? We know so much more about the effects of nutrition on health than was known when our grandparents were alive. Take advantage of all the research that's been done; otherwise, many scientists have been wasting their time all these years.

It's a Matter of Time

Did you ever think about how much time you assign to each of the daily tasks you do? If breakfast takes about 20 to 30 minutes and lunch 30 to 40 minutes and dinner 60 to 90 minutes, that's almost 3 hours a day spent eating. Let's now add another 60 minutes a day for exercising, and maybe 30 minutes for something to de-stress you, like meditation, aromatherapy, or yoga. You're up to four hours a day spent entirely on you and your health. Now, let's say you take 30 minutes to get ready for work, spend 8 hours a day working, and waste 1 hour commuting. (I know, you only wish it were so little with the traffic on the freeways these days!) We're up to a little over 13 hours. If you spend another 30 minutes showering, and you get a good night's sleep of 8 hours, you've used up about 22 hours of the day so far. You still get two hours to do anything you want. So don't tell me, or worse, yourself, that you don't have time to do what it takes to be healthy. Again, though, it does come down to choices. Consider that, out of a 24-hour day, you use 4 hours or 17 percent to be healthy; that doesn't seem like much. To know that you're doing something good for yourself is mentally uplifting. To see the results is like "icing on the cake."

Boomers have been dubbed the "me" generation. I believe with that thinking has come the demand that everything should happen immediately. No waiting for food—we have fast-food restaurants. No waiting for making a bank deposit—we have drive-up windows. The desire for instant gratification has prompted many boomers to try whatever quick-fix method comes aboard the diet bandwagon. Let's get one thing straight. There is no quick fix. Accept it and deal with the slow process of taking the weight off, which, by the way, didn't get put on overnight either. If you can't be patient with the process, you'll never make it to your goal. And if you're not diligent about policing yourself (others can't do it for you), all your efforts will be for naught.

Setting Limits

Let's say that you've lost the weight and are feeling really good about yourself. You have more energy than you've had in a long time and you've dropped a couple of clothes sizes. You can't believe you finally did it, but the proof is there. Now how do you keep the weight off "for good"?

You have to set limits. Your credit card has spending limits. Roads and highways have speed limits. In the same way, your weight should have limits. You may be the type who's willing to buy things on credit and drive faster than the speed limit (always looking in your rearview mirror!), but when it comes to your weight, there shouldn't be any breaking of the laws. There's a consequence for everything you do wrong. Go over your credit limit and you get high interest payments. Go over the speed limit and you get a ticket. Go over your "feed limit" and you're back to dieting.

I suppose the greatest anomaly to me is seeing people do what it takes to lose weight, and then allow themselves to regain it. If losing weight was important enough to you, and you feel better because you lost the weight, why would you allow anything or anyone, especially yourself, to sabotage your efforts? So, my question to you is—how many pounds do you think you should allow yourself to gain back before you put the brakes on? Natural water retention at various times may show up as 2 to 3 pounds on the scale. Then maybe a couple of pounds creeps back on because you've not been eating properly. So let's agree that you get a 5-pound window before you must take corrective action.

If you've been following the Choice Plan, then go back to tracking. If you've been doing the Portion-Control Plan, then measure what you're eating. Whatever method you used to lose weight, go back to it and refresh your skills. It may take some time for you to make these approaches a part of you, where you know instinctively when you're straying. **Just don't give up!** To paraphrase an old Tibetan saying, "Failing to practice what you've learned is like turning the lights on and then shutting your eyes."

The bathroom scale and your clothes will be your best guide. I previously recommended that while you are losing weight, you weigh yourself only once a week. At this point, you can either continue with that approach or consider weighing yourself every other week or even just once a month. You may never be free from monitoring, unless you can actually sense when you're starting to gain. To use myself as an example, I can put my hands on my waist and know when I've put on a pound or two. In fact, I sometimes challenge myself to estimate whether I've gained any weight by first feeling my waist, taking a guess at how much, and then getting on the scale to see whether I'm right. After you've done this a number of times, you get more in tune with how you feel and what your body looks like, without even needing to see the exact numbers on a scale.

Looking Within

There's nothing wrong in looking for help on your journey. That's why Dorothy, in *The Wizard of Oz,* went to the Emerald City to consult the Wizard. She figured (or hoped) that he would have the answers. I hope that this book will be the inspiration for you. Yet, as Dorothy found out from Glenda, the Good Witch of the North, you've always had the power within you to succeed. You just have to find out for yourself.

Do you remember seeing *The Wizard of Oz* for the first time? It started out as a black-and-white movie and then, when Dorothy lands in Oz and steps out of her house, the scene opens up in color. Every time I see that movie, I'm still moved by the feeling of going from drab black and white to spectacular color. That's the feeling I'd like you to have as you lose weight. To have a sense of a brighter tomorrow, feeling better, having more energy, fitting into your clothes (even buying some new ones), and just feeling good about yourself.

I'd love to hear from you—tell me of your weight-loss success stories, and what it was that made the difference for you. You can reach me by e-mail at roberta@advantagediets.com or write me at PO Box 83, Lynnwood, WA 98046-0083. My phone number is 1-425-778-1340 if you'd like to talk.

Good luck on your journey!

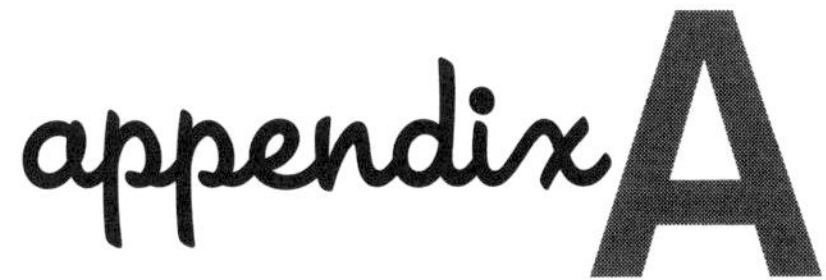

Fiber Choices

Fruits

Fruit	Amount	Fiber
Raspberries	1 cup	6 grams
Prunes, dried	4	4 grams
Banana	1 small	3 grams
Apple	1	3 grams
Orange	1	2 grams
Peach	1	1 gram

Vegetables

Vegetable	Amount	Fiber
Acorn squash	3/4 cup	4 grams
Brussels sprouts	1/2 cup	3 grams
Cabbage	1/2 cup	2 grams
Carrot	1	2 grams
Potato, peeled	1	2 grams
Tomato	1	2 grams
Asparagus	1/2 cup	1 gram
Broccoli	1/2 cup	1 gram
Cauliflower	1/2 cup	1 gram
Romaine lettuce	1 cup	1 gram
Spinach	1/2 cup	1 gram
Zucchini	1 cup	1 gram

Starchy Vegetables

Vegetable	Amount	Fiber
Black-eyed peas	1/2 cup	4 grams
Lima beans	1/2 cup	4 grams
Kidney beans	1/2 cup	3 grams

Grains

Grain	Amount	Fiber
Brown rice	1 cup	3 grams
Oatmeal	2/3 cup	3 grams
Whole wheat cereal	1 cup	3 grams
Whole wheat bread	1 slice	2 grams
White rice	1 cup	1 gram

Source: National Institutes of Health Digestive Diseases

Sample Fiber Menu

Food	Quantity	Fiber Content
Breakfast		
Raisin Bran cereal	1 cup	5 grams
Banana	1 medium	2 grams
1 cup low-fat or skim milk		
Lunch		
Turkey sandwich with whole-wheat bread, lettuce, and tomatoes	2 slices bread 1/2 tomato	4 grams 1 gram
Mixed raw vegetables (carrot sticks, cauliflower, celery, green beans)	1/2 cup	3 grams
Apple	1/2 cup	3 grams
Dinner		
Grilled chicken breast		
Sautéed cabbage	1 cup	2 grams
Brown rice and lentils	1/2 cup	5 grams
Stewed prunes	1/3 cup	3 grams
Total		**28 grams**

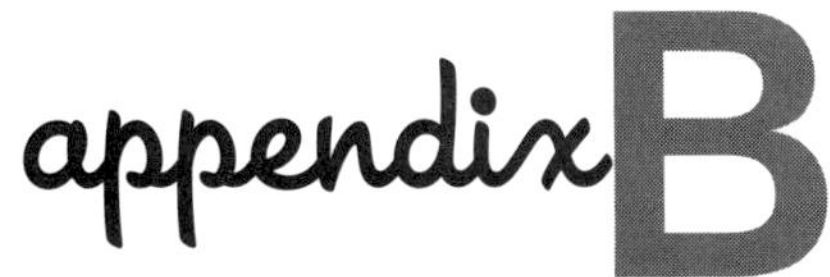

Comparison of Fats

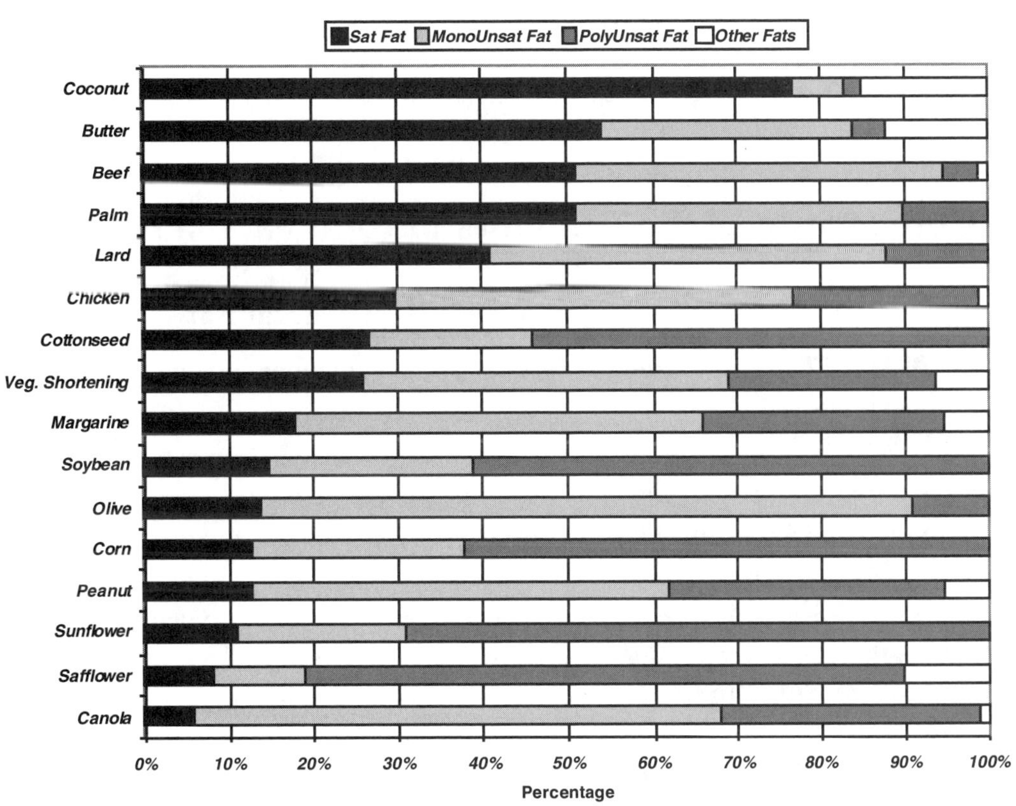

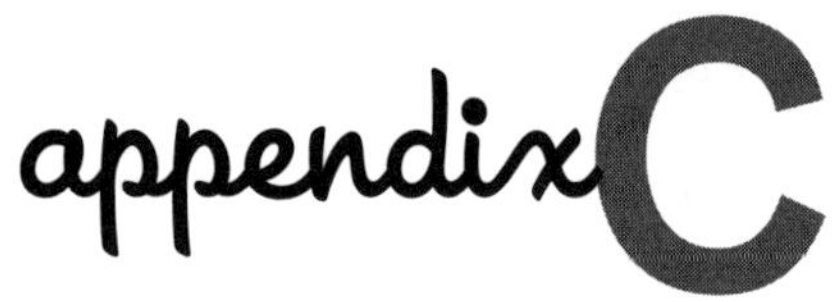

How Much Fat Is in Your Food

Find out how many teaspoons fat are in some of the foods you eat. When you look at a food label, you can calculate how many teaspoons of fat are in the food by dividing the grams of total fat by five.

Comparison of the Amounts of Total Fats in Foods

	Number of Teaspoons Total Fat
Fat (1 teaspoon):	**1**
Butter, oil, lard	
Milk (8 oz.):	
1%	0.5
2%	1
Whole	2
Low-Fat Cheese (1 oz.):	**0.5**
Cottage (low-fat—1/4 cup), feta, mozzarella, ricotta	
Medium-Fat Cheese (1 oz.):	**1**
Cottage (4.5%—1/4 cup), feta, mozzarella, ricotta	
High-Fat Cheese (1 oz.):	**1.5**
American, cheddar, Monterey, Muenster, Parmesan, Swiss	
Very Lean Meat (3 oz.):	**1**
Poultry: without skin *Fish:* cod, flounder, haddock, halibut, trout, tuna in water *Misc.:* one egg, 4 oz. tofu, 1/4 cup egg substitute	
Lean Meat (3 oz.):	**2**
Beef: round, sirloin, flank, tenderloin *Fish:* oysters, salmon, sardines, tuna in oil (drained) *Pork:* ham, center loin chop *Poultry:* with skin	

	Number of Teaspoons Total Fat
Medium-Fat Meat (3 oz.):	**3**
Beef: ground beef, corned beef, short ribs, "prime cuts"	
Fish: fried	
Lamb: rib roast, ground	
Pork: top loin, chop Boston, cutlet	
Poultry: dark meat with skin, ground, fried	
High-Fat Meat (3 oz.):	**5**
Polish sausage, spareribs, hot dog, processed sandwich meats	

Amount of Fat in Fast-Food Restaurant Selections

	Number of Teaspoons Total Fat
McDonald's	
McDonald's Double Quarter-Pounder with Extra Cheese	10
Big Mac	7
Double Cheeseburger	5.5
Cheeseburger	3
Large French Fries	5
Burger King	
Original Double Whopper with Cheese	14
Original Whopper with Cheese	10
Original Whopper	9
Cheeseburger	3.5
Large French Fries	5
Pizza Hut	
Super Supreme (per slice)	3
Chicken Supreme (per slice)	1.5

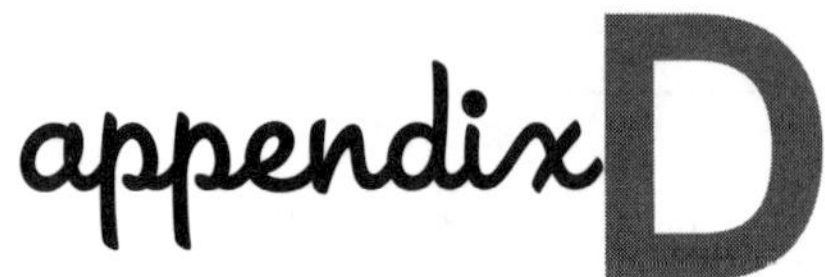

How Much Sugar Is in Your Food

Find out how many teaspoons sugar are in some of the foods you eat. When you look at a food label, you can calculate how many teaspoons sugar are in the food by dividing the grams of sugar by 4. Keep in mind that those sugars can be naturally occurring or added.

Sugar in Our Food

Food	Quantity	Number of Teaspoons Sugar
Apple pie	1/8 pie	5
Brownies	1 to 3 inches square	5
Cheesecake	1 slice	6
Chocolate bar	1 1/2 ounces	6
Chocolate-chip cookie	1 to 4 inches diameter	4
Chocolate syrup	1 tablespoon	5
Fruit punch	8 ounces	7
Gelatin dessert	1/2 cup	3
Gum drops	10 small	7
Ice cream	1/2 cup	5
Pudding	1/2 cup	6
Soft drinks	12 ounces	10
Spaghetti sauce	1 cup	3
Sugared cereal	3/4 cup	3

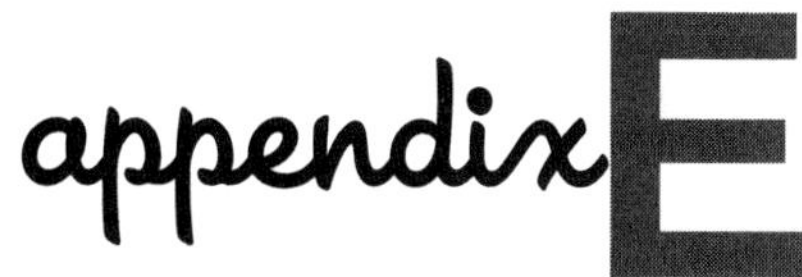

Weight-Loss Log

Goal Weight: ______________________

Date	Weight	Gain (+) / Loss (–) from Last Weigh-In	Number of Pounds to Reach Goal Weight

Portion-Control Logs

Portion-Control Log—My Usual Amounts

Date: ________

Meal	Food	Amount (Ounces, Cups)	Standard Serving Size

Portion-Control Log—One-Half My Usual Amounts

Date: ________

Meal	Food	Original Amount (Ounces, Cups)	Half Original Amount (Ounces, Cups)	Standard Serving Size

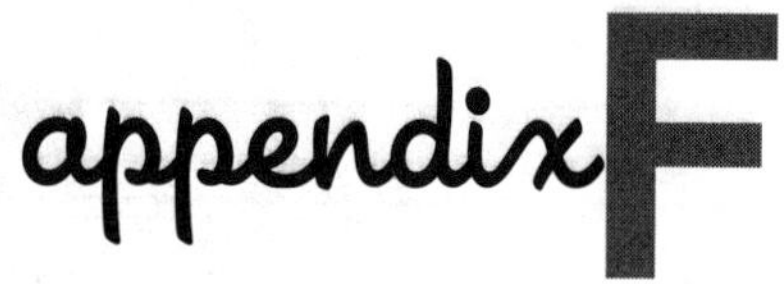

Hunger-Fullness Gauge

If you want to keep track of how responsive you are to hunger and fullness signs, use the following gauges. Make copies as you need them. I've included an example for you. Use a hollow arrow to note when you start eating and a black arrow to show when you stop.

Date ____________ Meal ____________

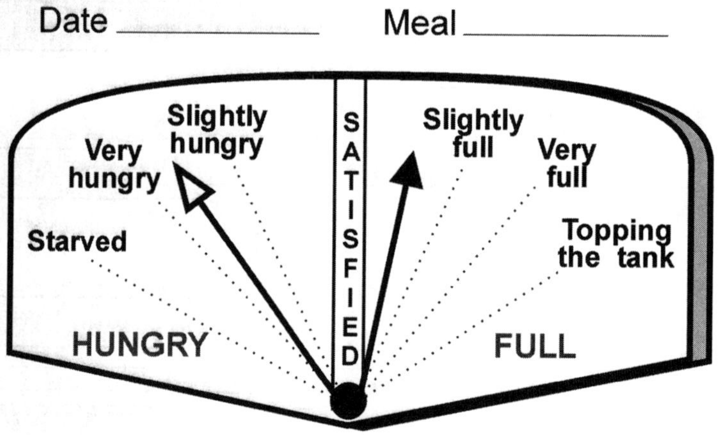

© 1999 HealthPro. All rights reserved.

Hunger-Fullness Gauge

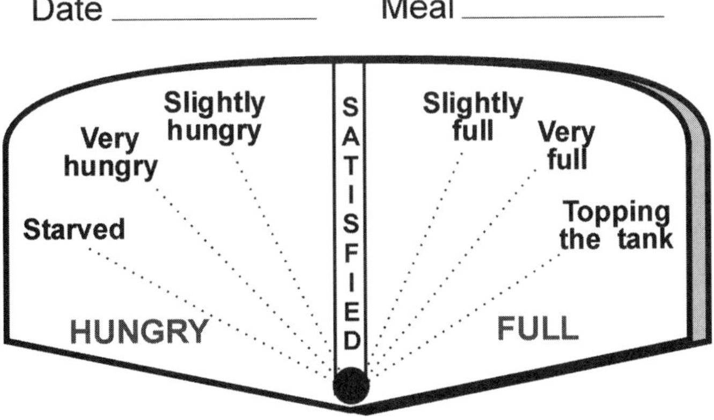

© 1999 HealthPro. All rights reserved.

Date ____________ Meal ____________

Slightly hungry
Very hungry
Starved
HUNGRY
SATISFIED
Slightly full
Very full
Topping the tank
FULL

© 1999 HealthPro. All rights reserved.

Date ____________ Meal ____________

Slightly hungry
Very hungry
Starved
HUNGRY
SATISFIED
Slightly full
Very full
Topping the tank
FULL

© 1999 HealthPro. All rights reserved.

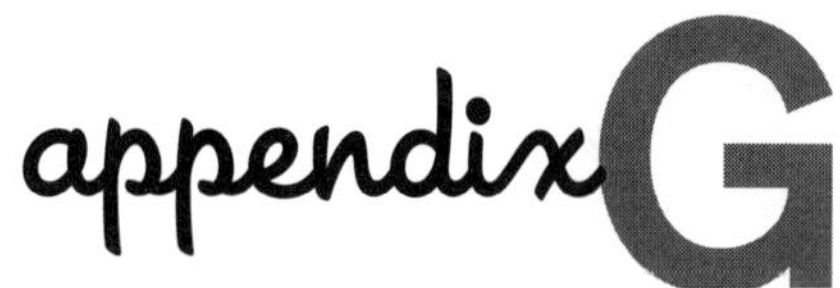

Choice Tracker

THE CHOICE PLAN

Date ________ Plan ________________ Calories ________

STARCH	VEG	FRUIT	DRY BEANS LEGUMES	MILK	MEAT: EGGS, CHEESE & NUTS	MEAT: MEAT & POULTRY	MEAT: FISH	FAT	SWEETS
○	△	□	☾	⬭	◇	◇	◇	⬡	💧
○	△	□	☾	⬭	◇	◇	◇	⬡	💧
○	△	□		⬭	◇	◇	◇	⬡	
○	△	□			◇	◇	◇	⬡	
○	△				◇	◇	◇	⬡	
○	△				◇	◇	◇	⬡	
○	△				◇	◇	◇	⬡	
○					◇	◇	◇	⬡	
○								⬡	

Don't forget your liquids. Put an "x" in a box each time you have 8 ounces of water or some other beverage.

Water or beverage	8 oz.	8 oz.	8 oz.	8 oz.	8 oz.	8 oz.	8 oz.	8 oz.

©2001 Advantage Diets - All rights reserved.

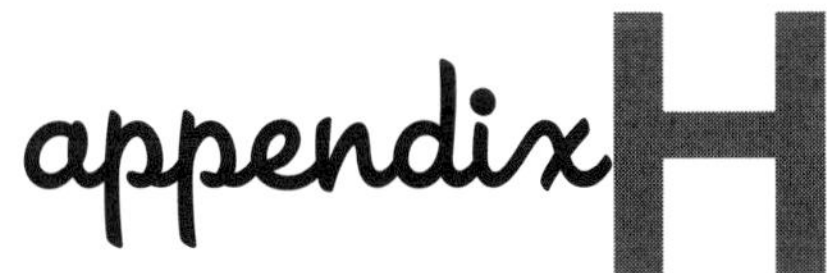

Food List

It is impossible to provide all the foods you might ever eat. If a particular food is not included here, try to find something that is similar to it. You may have to look up the separate ingredients for a dish and track those individually. If you're dining out, ask how the dish is prepared.

Food	Amt.	Starch	Veg.	Fruit	Beans/ Legumes	Milk	Meat	Fat	Sweets
Alcohol Beverages									
Beer	12 oz.	1						2	
Light beer	12 oz.							2	
Gin, rum, scotch, vodka, whiskey	1½ oz.							2	
Wine	4 oz.							2	
Beans, Peas, and Lentils (Cooked)									
Baked beans	½ cup				1				
Beans (garbanzo, kidney, navy, pinto)	½ cup				1				
Lima beans	⅔ cup				1				
Lentils	½ cup				1				
Refried beans (low fat)	½ cup				1			1	
Split peas (yellow, green)	½ cup				1				
Breads									
Bagel	1	2							
Biscuits	1 small	1						1	
Blueberry muffin	1 small	1½						1	

Food	Amt.	Starch	Veg.	Fruit	Beans/ Legumes	Milk	Meat	Fat	Sweets
Bread (white, whole wheat)	1 slice	1							
Bread sticks, 4 in. long × 1/2 in.	2 sticks	1							
Bread stuffing mix, prepared	1/2 cup	1 1/2						1 1/2	
Cornbread, 3-in. square	1	1						1	
Croutons, baked	1 cup	1							
English muffins	1	2							
French toast, prepared	2 slices	2					1/2	1/2	
Hamburger or hot dog bun	1	2							
Pancakes, 4 in. across	3	2						1	
Pita, 6 in. across	1	2							
Roll, plain	1 small	1							
Sweet roll or Danish	1							2	2 1/2
Tortilla, 6 to 7 in. across	1	1							
Waffle, 4 in. square	1	1							
Cakes, Doughnuts, Pies, and Puddings									
Angel food cake, 1/2 cake	1 slice								2
Brownie, 2-in. square	1							1	1
Cake, frosted, 1/8 cake	1 slice							1 1/2	2
Cake, unfrosted, 1/8 cake								1	1
Carrot cake, 2-in. square	1							2	2
Cheesecake, 1/10 cake	1 slice							5	2
Chocolate cake, 1/8 cake	1							2	3
Cupcake, frosted	1 small							1	2
Doughnut, plain cake, medium	1							2	1 1/2
Doughnut, glazed 3 3/4 in.	1							2	2
Fruitcake	1 slice							1/2	2

Food	Amt.	Starch	Veg.	Fruit	Beans/ Legumes	Milk	Meat	Fat	Sweets
Gelatin, regular	½ cup								1
Pie, fruit, 2 crusts, ⅙ pie	1 slice							2	3
Pie, pumpkin or custard, ⅛ pie	1 slice							2	1
Pound cake	1 slice							2	2½
Pudding (low-fat milk)	½ cup								2
Pudding (sugar-free, low-fat milk)	½ cup								1
Toaster pastry	1							1	2
Candy									
Chocolate	1 oz.							2	1
Chocolate mints	5							1	2
Fruit leather	¾ oz.								1
Hard candy	2								1
Jelly beans	15								2½
Marshmallows	4								1½
Cereals and Grains									
Cereals, cold or hot	¾ cup	1							
Cornmeal (dry)	3 TB.	1							
Couscous, cooked	⅓ cup	1							
Flour (dry)	3 TB.	1							
Granola, low fat	¼ cup	1							
Grits	½ cup	1							
Muesli	¼ cup	1							
Oats and oatmeal	¾ cup	1							
Pasta, cooked	½ cup	1							
Puffed cereal	1½ cups	1							
Rice (white, brown), cooked	½ cup	1							
Wheat germ	3 TB.	1							

Food	Amt.	Starch	Veg.	Fruit	Beans/ Legumes	Milk	Meat	Fat	Sweets
				Cheese					
American	1 oz.						1	1	
Brie	1 oz.						1	1	
Cheddar	1 oz.						1	1	
Cheese, fat free	1 oz.						1		
Cottage cheese (skim, low fat)	1/4 cup						1		
Cream cheese, low fat	2 TB.							1	
Cream cheese, regular	1 TB.							1	
Feta	1 oz.						1	1/2	
Goat	1 oz.						1	1	
Monterey Jack	1 oz.						1	1	
Mozzarella	1 oz.						1	1/2	
Parmesan, grated	2 TB.						1		
Ricotta	1 oz.						1	1	
Swiss	1 oz.						1	1	
				Chips, Crackers, and Snacks					
Corn chips	1 oz.	1						2	
Potato chips	1 oz.	1						2	
Popcorn, air-popped	3 cups	1							
Tortilla chips	1 oz.	1						2	
Animal crackers	8	1							
Graham cracker, 2 1/2-in. square	3	1							
Matzo	3/4 oz.	1							
Melba toast	4 slices	1							
Oyster crackers	24 items	1							
Pretzels	3/4 oz.	1							
Rice cakes, 4 in. across	2	1							
Saltine-type crackers	6	1							
Snack chips, fat free (3/4 oz.)		15–20	1						
Wheat crackers	7	1						1	

Food	Amt.	Starch	Veg.	Fruit	Beans/ Legumes	Milk	Meat	Fat	Sweets
Combination Dishes									
Beef stew	1 cup	1	1/2				3	1	
Beef tamale pie	1	1 1/2					2	2	
Burrito with meat	1 small	1 1/2					2	1	
Cheese pizza	1 slice	1					1	2	
Chicken pot pie	1	1 1/2					2 1/2	2	
Chili con carne	1 cup				2		1/2	2	
Chow mein (chicken, beef, pork)	2 cups	2	1				2	1	
Corned beef hash	1 cup	1 1/2					2	3 1/2	
Egg roll	1	1	1				1		
Enchiladas, beef	1	1 1/2					2	1	
Lasagna with meat	1 cup	1 1/2					2	2	
Macaroni and cheese	2/3 cup	1 1/2					2	4	
Meat knish	1	1					2	1	
Pepperoni pizza	1 slice	1					1	2	
Pork tamales	1	1/2					1	2 1/2	
Quesadillas	1	1					2	2	
Shrimp creole with rice	1 cup	1	1				3		
Shrimp egg roll	2	1 1/2					1/2	1 1/2	
Spaghetti in sauce	1 cup	2						1	
Spanakopitta	1 cup	1					1	4	
Cookies									
Chocolate-chip cookie	1							1 1/2	1
Cookie, filled sandwich	1							1	1
Fig bar	2								1 1/2
Gingersnaps	3								1
Granola bar	1 bar							1	1
Vanilla wafers	5							1	1
Whole-wheat crackers, no fat added (3/4 oz.)	2–5	1							

Food	Amt.	Starch	Veg.	Fruit	Beans/ Legumes	Milk	Meat	Fat	Sweets
Dairy									
Cream, half-and-half	2 TB.							1	
Cream, whipping	1 TB.							1	
Milk, 1%	1 cup					1			
Milk, 2%	1 cup					1		1	
Milk, chocolate, whole milk	1 cup					1		1	1
Milk, skim	1 cup					1			
Milk, whole	1 cup					1		1½	
Sour cream	2 TB.							2	
Yogurt, low fat, fruit	1 cup	3				1			
Yogurt, low fat, plain	¾ cup					1			
Yogurt, fat free, plain	¾ cup					1			
Dressings, Fats, Oils, Sauces, and Spreads									
Butter	1 tsp.							1	
Caesar dressing	2 TB.							3	
Cocktail sauce	¼ cup								1
Guacamole	2 TB.							1	
Italian dressing	2 TB.							2	
Jam or jelly	1 TB.								1
Margarine	1 tsp.							1	
Margarine, low fat	1 TB.							1	
Mayonnaise	1 tsp.							1	
Mayonnaise, low fat	1 TB.							1	
Oil—monounsaturated (olive, canola, peanut)	1 tsp.							1	
Oil—polyunsaturated (corn, safflower, soybean)	1 tsp.							1	
Ranch dressing	2 TB.							3	
Salad dressing, fat free	¼ cup	1							

Food	Amt.	Starch	Veg.	Fruit	Beans/ Legumes	Milk	Meat	Fat	Sweets
Shortening	1 tsp.							1	
Syrup, regular	1 TB.								1
Thousand Island dressing	2 TB.							2½	
Frozen Desserts									
Fruit juice bar, 100% juice	1 bar								1
Ice cream	½ cup							2	1
Ice cream, fat free, sugar free	½ cup								1
Ice cream, light	½ cup							1	1
Sherbet, sorbet	½ cup								2
Yogurt, frozen, low fat, fat free	⅓ cup								1
Fruits									
Canned in juice or light syrup	½ cup			1					
Dried	¼ cup			1					
Fresh, small to medium	1			1					
Juice or nectar	½ cup			1					
Apple, small	1			1					
Applesauce, unsweetened	½ cup			1					
Apricot, dried	8 halves			1					
Apricot, fresh	4 whole			1					
Banana, small	1			1					
Blackberries, blueberries	¾ cup			1					
Dates	3			1					
Figs, dried	1½			1					
Figs, fresh	2			1					
Fruit cocktail	½ cup			1					

Food	Amt.	Starch	Veg.	Fruit	Beans/ Legumes	Milk	Meat	Fat	Sweets
Fruit, canned, light syrup	1/2 cup			1					
Grapefruit, large	1/2			1					
Grapes	17			1					
Melon	1/2 cup			1					
Orange, small	1			1					
Peach, medium, fresh	1			1					
Pear, large, fresh	1			1					
Pineapple, fresh	3/4 cup			1					
Prunes, dried	3			1					
Raisins	2 TB.			1					
Raspberries	1 cup			1					
Strawberries, whole	1 1/2 cup			1					
Meats, Eggs, and Nuts									
Lean Cuts									
Beef, select or choice, trimmed (round, sirloin, flank, tenderloin, roast, steak, ground round)	3 oz.						3		
Lamb (roast, chop, leg)	3 oz.						3		
Pork, lean (ham, Canadian bacon, tenderloin, center loin chop)	3 oz.						3		
Veal (lean chop, roast)	3 oz.						3		
Medium-Fat Cuts									
Beef (ground, meatloaf, corned, short ribs, prime grades)	3 oz.						3	1	
Lamb (rib roast, ground)	3 oz.						3	1	
Pork (top loin, chop, Boston butt, cutlet)	3 oz.						3	1	
Tofu	4 oz.						1	1/2	

Food	Amt.	Starch	Veg.	Fruit	Beans/ Legumes	Milk	Meat	Fat	Sweets
High-Fat Cuts									
Deli meats (bologna, salami)	1 oz.						1	1	
Hot dog (beef, pork, combination)	2 oz.						1	2	
Pork (spareribs, ground, sausage, bacon)	3 oz.						3	3	
Eggs									
Egg, raw, large	1						1	1/2	
Egg substitute, cooked	1/4 cup						1	1/2	
Omelet, cheese (1 egg)	1						1	1 1/2	
Scrambled eggs	1/4 cup						1	1/2	
Nuts and Seeds									
Flaxseed	3 TB.						1	1	
Nut butters (almond, cashew, peanut)	2 TB.						1	1	
Nuts (almonds, cashews, peanuts, pecans, pistachio)	1/4 cup						1	3	
Seeds (pumpkin, sesame, sunflower)	3 TB.						2	2	
Tahini	2 tsp.							1	
Poultry									
Dark meat, w/o skin	3 oz.						3	1	
Fried	3 oz.						3	2	
Ground	3 oz.						3	1	
White meat, w/o skin	3 oz.						3		

Food	Amt.	Starch	Veg.	Fruit	Beans/ Legumes	Milk	Meat	Fat	Sweets
				Seafood					
Cod, flounder, haddock, halibut, tuna (fresh or canned in water)	3 oz.						3		
Crab, steamed, meat only	3 oz.						3		
Fried fish	3 oz.						3	2	
Herring	1 oz.						3		
Salmon, canned or fresh	3 oz.						3		
Shrimp	3 oz.						3		
Tuna, canned in oil	3 oz.						3	1	
				Vegetables					
All except starchy, cooked	½ cup		1						
All except starchy, raw	1 cup		1						
				Vegetables—Starchy					
Corn	½ cup	1							
Corn on cob, medium	1	1							
Peas, green	½ cup	1							
Potato, baked or boiled	1 small	1							
Potato, mashed	½ cup	1							
Squash, winter (sweet, acorn, butternut)	1 cup	1							
Yam, sweet potato, plain	½ cup	1							

Nutrition data provided by Nutritionist Pro software from First DataBank.

For more food lists, contact the American Diabetes Association or see Exchanges for All Occasions by Marion Franz, R.D., M.S. (International Diabetes Center, 2000).

appendix

% Daily Value Converter

% Daily Value is the portion of your daily nutrient needs supplied by the food. The % Daily Values listed on the label are for a 2,000-calorie diet. If you eat more or fewer than 2,000 calories a day, the converter on the next page adjusts the % Daily Values to your calorie level.

How to Use the % Daily Value Converter:

In the first column, find the % Daily Value listed on the label for any nutrient (except cholesterol and sodium, which have the same % Daily Value as on the label for all calorie levels).

Run your finger across that row until you come to the column with your calorie needs.

The number you see there is your adjusted % Daily Value for your calorie level.

Daily Values for Different Calorie Levels

Calories	Total Fat (g)	Saturated Fat (g)	Fiber (g)*	Protein (g)
1,200	40	16	20	46**
1,400	47	16	20	46**
1,600	53	17	20	46**
1,800	60	20	21	46**
2,000 Reference Diet	65	21	25	50
2,200	73	24	25	55
2,500	80	25	30	65

** 20 grams is the minimum amount of fiber recommended for all calorie levels below 2,000. Source: National Cancer Institute.*

*** 46 grams is the minimum amount of protein recommended for all calorie levels below 1,800. Source: Recommended Dietary Allowances, 1989.*

The following table shows you Daily Values for the important nutrients.

% Daily Value Converter

Daily Value Listed on the Label	Calories % 1200	1500	1800	2200	2500
	Adjusted % Daily Value				
1%	2	1	1	1	1
2%	3	3	2	2	2
3%	5	4	3	3	2
4%	7	5	4	4	3
5%	8	7	6	5	4
6%	10	8	7	5	5
7%	12	9	8	6	6
8%	13	11	9	7	6
9%	15	12	10	8	7
10%	17	13	11	9	8
11%	18	15	12	10	9
12%	20	16	13	11	10
13%	22	17	14	12	10
14%	23	19	16	13	11
15%	25	20	17	14	12
16%	27	21	18	15	13
17%	28	23	19	15	14
18%	30	24	20	16	14
19%	32	25	21	17	15
20%	33	27	22	18	16
21%	35	28	23	19	17
22%	37	29	24	20	18
23%	38	31	26	21	18
24%	40	32	27	22	19
25%	42	33	28	23	20
26%	43	35	29	24	21
27%	45	36	30	25	22
28%	46	37	31	25	22
29%	48	39	32	26	23
30%	50	40	33	27	24
31%	51	41	34	28	25
32%	53	43	36	29	26
33%	55	44	37	30	26
34%	56	45	38	31	27
35%	58	47	39	32	28

© 1996 HealthPro. All rights reserved.

appendix J

Additives

Acesulfame K (acesulfame potassium) is an artificial sweetener. Used in chewing gum, diet soft drinks, frozen desserts, gelatins, baked goods, tabletop sweeteners.

Alginates come from seaweed and are used for their gelatinous properties as stabilizers in frozen desserts, baked goods, candies, icings, cheese spreads, and salad dressings.

Aluminum sulfate has a slight astringent taste and is used in pickles.

Butylated hydroxyanisole (BHA) and **butylated hydroxytoluene (BHT)** are preservatives and antioxidants used in many products from beverages to frozen desserts, cereals, and shortening. They are used to prevent fats and oils in foods from becoming rancid.

Calcium propionate and sodium propionate are preservatives used to inhibit mold growth on breads and rolls.

Carrageenan comes from seaweed and is used as a stabilizing and thickening agent. It's used in many products such as frozen desserts, chocolate milk, and jelly.

EDTA (ethylenediaminetetraacetic acid) is a chelating agent that is added to foods to trap metal impurities that come from the processing of the food with metal equipment.

Food dyes are used so widely in beverages, candies, desserts, and baked goods that they may be hard to avoid. For some reason, many people are not accepting of foods in their natural color. For example, there isn't enough mint in mint ice cream to make it that bright green color. But people expect it, or maybe we've been trained to expect it.

Fumaric acid adds tartness to such products as gelatins and puddings.

Gums are gelling and thickening agents.

Hydrolyzed vegetable protein is a flavor enhancer that is often included in franks, stews, soups, and sauces.

Lecithin is an emulsifying agent for baked goods, frozen desserts, chocolate, and margarine. It keeps water and oil from separating, retards spoilage from fats going rancid, and makes cakes fluffier.

Mono- and diglycerides are emulsifiers used in baked goods, candy, margarine, and peanut butter. They help to make baked goods fluffier and to keep oil in margarine and peanut butter from separating out.

MSG (monosodium glutamate) is a flavor enhancer used in frozen entrées, dressings, soups, and restaurant foods. Some people are very sensitive to it. Many Chinese restaurants use a great deal of MSG. If you get reactions from MSG, request that your dish be made without it.

Phosphates act as buffers and emulsifiers and inhibit discoloration in baked goods, carbonated drinks, cereals, cheeses, and potato flakes.

Polysorbate 60 is an emulsifier in baked goods, frozen desserts, and imitation dairy products. It keeps bakery goods fresher longer, and keeps the oil in artificial whipped cream from separating.

Potassium bromate is a conditioning and bleaching agent for dough.

Propyl gallate is used as an antioxidant in foods to prevent fats and oils from going rancid.

Sodium benzoate is a preservative that prevents the growth of microorganisms in acidic foods such as carbonated drinks, fruit juice, pickles, and preserves.

Sodium nitrate and **sodium nitrite** are used to color, flavor, and preserve such foods as bacon, frankfurters, ham, and luncheon meats.

Sulfites are used in wines to prevent bacterial growth and on fruits, vegetables, and shrimp to keep them from browning or spotting. Look for words in the ingredient list that include *sulfur, sulfite, bisulfate,* and *metabisulfate.* In 1986, the FDA banned the use of sulfites on produce served at salad bars in restaurants or grocery stores because many people are allergic to the additive.

Appendix K

Exercise Log—Doing Your AFS

Week of ______________________

Date/Time	Flexibility Stretches		Strength Free Weights, Resistance, Floor Exercises		Aerobics	Endurance	
	Minutes	**Sets****	**Pounds***	**Sets****	**Exercises**	**Type**	**Minutes**
Sunday							
Monday							
Tuesday							
Wednesday							
Thursday							
Friday							
Saturday							

* *Write down the number of pounds in your weights.*

** *There are 10 reps (repetitions) per set.*

appendix L

Additional Resources

Ackerman, Diane. *A Natural History of the Senses.* New York: Vintage Books, 1990.

Baker, Dan, Ph.D. *What Happy People Know.* Emmaus, PA: Rodale, 2003.

Bridges, William. *Transitions.* Reading, MA: Addison-Wesley Publishing Company, 1980.

Bundy, Beverly. *The Century in Food.* Portland, OR: Collectors Press, 2002.

Clark, Nancy, M.S., R.D. *Nancy Clark's Sports Nutrition Guidebook.* Champaign, IL: Human Kinetics, 1997.

Heber, David, M.D., Ph.D. *What Color Is Your Diet?* New York: Regan Books, 2001.

Lappé, Frances Moore. *Diet for a Small Planet.* New York: Ballantine Books, 1975.

Pennington, Jean, Ph.D., et al. *Bowes & Church's Food Values of Portions Commonly Used, Seventeenth Edition.* Philadelphia: J.B. Lippincott Company, 1998.

Prochaska, James, Ph.D., John Norcross, Ph.D., and Carlo Diclemente, Ph.D. *Changing for Good.* New York: Avon Books, 1994.

Rolls, Barbara, Ph.D., and Robert A. Barnett. *The Volumetrics Weight-Control Plan.* New York: HarperTorch, 2000.

Schremp, Gerry. *Kitchen Culture.* New York: Pharos Books—A Scripps Howard Company, 1991.

Warshaw, Hope. *Guide to Healthy Restaurant Eating.* American Diabetes Association, 2002.

Weldon, Glen, ed. *Dietary Options for Cancer Survivors.* Washington, D.C.: American Institute for Cancer Research, 2002.

Wennik, Roberta Schwartz, M.S., R.D. *Beyond Food Labels.* New York: Perigee, 1996.

———. *Your Personality Prescription.* New York: Kensington Books, 1999.

Wurtman, Judith J., Ph.D. *Managing Your Mind and Mood Through Food.* New York. Harper & Row, 1986.

Government Sites

Eating Smart: A Nutrition Resource List for Consumers
www.nal.usda.gov/fnic/pubs/bibs/gen/eatsmart.html

Food and Nutrition Information Center
www.nal.usda.gov/fnic/etext/fnic.html

Food and Nutrition Information Center's Vegetarian Nutrition Resource List
www.nal.usda.gov/fnic/pubs/bibs/gen/vegetarian.htm

National Cancer Institute
cancer.gov

Nutrition.gov
www.nutrition.gov/home/index.php3

USDA Community Nutrition Map
www.barc.usda.gov/bhnrc/cnrg/cnmap.html?file=state53.htm

Other Websites

American Dietetic Association (ADA)
www.eatright.org

American Heart Association
www.americanheart.org/

American Institute for Cancer Research (AICR)
www.aicr.org

Center for Science in the Public Interest (CSPI)
www.cspinet.org

Consumer Corner
www.nal.usda.gov/fnic/consumersite

International Food Information Council (IFIC), Educational Booklets & Brochures section
ific.org/publications/brochures

NHLBI Publications for Patients and Public National Heart, Lung, and Blood Institute (NHLBI)
www.nhlbi.nih.gov/health/pubs/pub_gen.htm

Slow Food
www.slowfood.com

Vegetarian Resource Group
www.vrg.org

Tools for Checking Your Diet

Dietary Guidelines for Americans, 5th Edition, U.S. Department of Agriculture
www.health.gov/dietaryguidelines/dga2000/document/frontcover.htm (HTML version)

www.usda.gov/cnpp/DietGd.pdf (PDF version)

www.health.gov/dietaryguidelines/dga2000/document/summary/default.htm (one-page summary)

www.usda.gov/cnpp/Pubs/DG2000/DietGuidBrochure.pdf (PDF version)

The Food Guide Pyramid (USDA)
www.pueblo.gsa.gov/cic_text/food/food-pyramid/main.htm

How Much Are You Eating? Putting the Guidelines into Practice (USDA)
www.usda.gov/cnpp/Pubs/Brochures/index.htm

Interactive Healthy Eating Index (USDA)
147.208.9.133

USDA Nutrient Database for Standard Reference
www.nal.usda.gov/fnic/cgi-bin/nut_search.pl

Search Engines

Nutrition Navigator
Tufts University Center on Nutrition Communication
navigator.tufts.edu

MEDLINEplus
medlineplus.gov
Healthfinder U.S. Department of Health and Human Services
www.healthfinder.gov

Health Information On-Line Food and Drug Administration
www.cfsan.fda.gov/~dms/fdonline.html

Newsletters

American Institute for Cancer Research Newsletter
aicr.donortrust.com/consumerpublications.asp?item=consumernews

Environmental Nutrition
www.environmentalnutrition.com

FDA Consumer
www.fda.gov/fdac

Food Reflections
lancaster.unl.edu/food/foodtalk.htm

Loma Linda University Vegetarian Nutrition & Health Letter
www.llu.edu/llu/vegetarian

Nutrition Action Healthletter
www.cspinet.org/nah

Nutrition Spotlight
www.oznet.ksu.edu/dp_fnut/spotlight/welcome.htm

Tufts Health & Nutrition Letter
healthletter.tufts.edu

University of California at Berkeley Wellness Letter
www.berkeleywellness.com

Recipe Sites

Stay Young at Heart—Cooking the Heart Healthy Way
www.nhlbi.nih.gov/health/public/heart/other/syah/index.htm

Delicious Decisions—American Heart Association
www.deliciousdecisions.org/

Meals for You
www.mealsforyou.com

About Produce
www.aboutproduce.com

American Institute of Cancer Research
www.aicr.org

America's Test Kitchen from the editors of Cook's Illustrated
www.americastestkitchen.com

What You Need to Know About … Busy Cooks
busycooks.about.com

Favorite Brand Name Recipes
www.favoritebrandrecipes.com

Food and Health Communications
www.foodandhealth.com/recipes.php

Food Network.com
www.foodtv.com

Fast-Food Nutrition Facts

Arby's
www.arbys.com/arb06.html

Burger King
www.burgerking.com/Food/nutrition/interactivewizard

McDonald's
www.mcdonalds.com/countries/usa/food

Pizza Hut
www.pizzahut.com/Nutrition

Quiznos Sub
www.quiznos.com

Subway
www.subway.com

Taco Bell
www.yum.com/nutrition/tb/nutrition_index.asp

Wendy's
www.wendys.com/w-4-3.shtml

All Fast Food Restaurants
www.fatcalories.com

index

D

G

H

I

J

K–L

M

N

O

P

Y–Z

The times, they are a-changin'

The *Boomer's Guide* series offers practical knowledge and advice about the really important things in life, geared specifically to the needs of baby boomers. You know—those of us now 40- or 50-something who have teen- or college-age children, aging parents, maturing marriages (or perhaps a new single status), looming retirement, investment and property responsibilities, new health and fitness concerns, and a realization that we are finally becoming our parents.

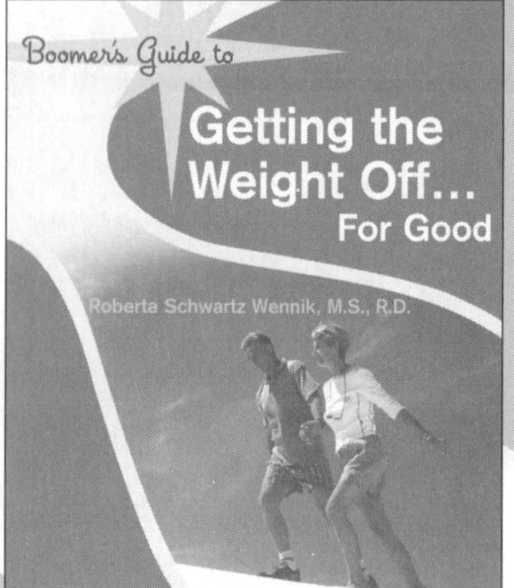

1-59257-160-3 • $16.95

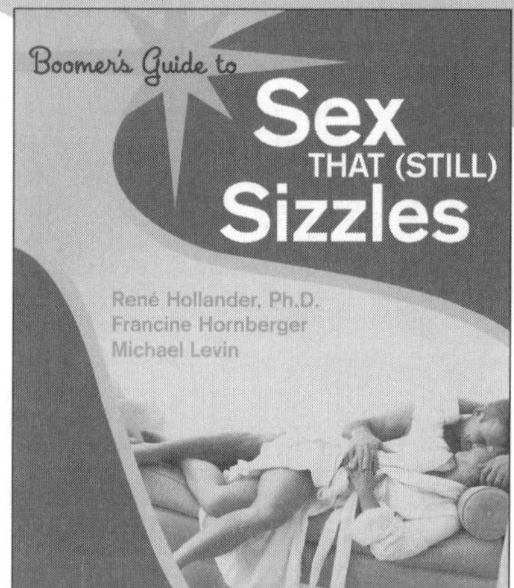

1-59257-155-7 • $16.95

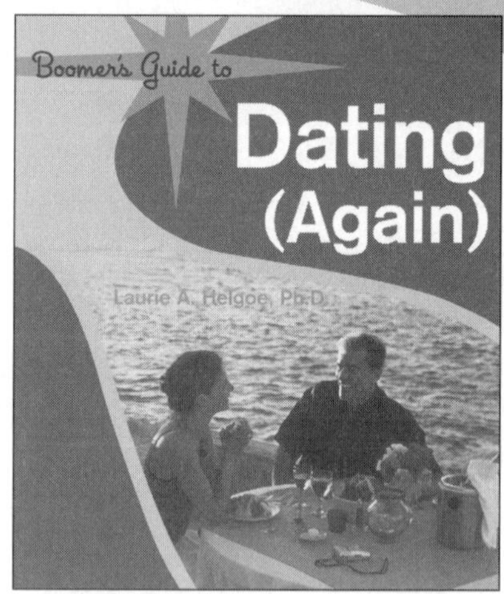

1-59257-164-6 • $16.95

Coming Summer of 2004:

Boomer's Guide to

Divorce

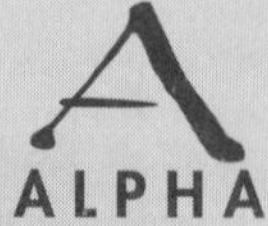

From the publishers of *The Complete Idiot's Guide*® series

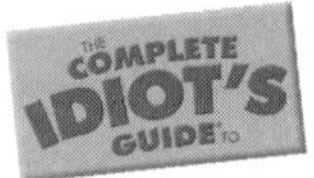